2014

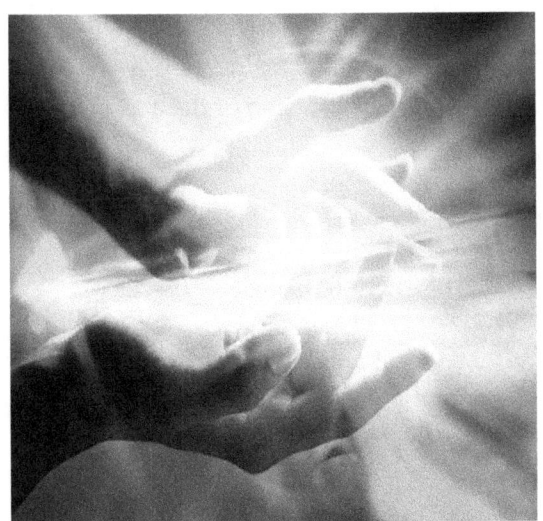

From Illness to **Wellness!**

From Illness to Wellness is based on a real life story of Dr. Guru, who has transformed his life from illness to wellness, through the simple & profound Vedic healing methods of India.

From Illness to Wellness!!!

All rights reserved. No parts of this publication may be reproduced, stored in a retrieval system, or transmitted, in any form or by any means, electronic, mechanical, photocopying, recording, or otherwise, without the prior permission of the author.

© Jay Kay 2014

ISBN 9781502704689
Published by
Jay Kay
writerjaykay@gmail.com

From Illness to Wellness!!!

Preface

From Illness to Wellness describes profound vedic healing method of Siddhic tradition. This compilation is based on a true story of transformation of Dr. Guru & research conducted by the World Health Organization (WHO), US. It's a holistic healing method, with profound wisdom of the East, and the West.

The profound **'HEALING METHODS'** techniques discussed in this book is an altruistic view of healing, and a contemporary therapy. This will lay foundations with a paradigm shift in the therapy treatments & holistic healing. What is the purpose of life without taking care of body?. The lack of awareness will result in diseases in body with conflicting mind in a state of despair. Today, the World is haunted by false diseases, which are false disorders of the mind, and body, whilst your body has the intelligence to build the defense mechanism as needed.

I'd like to invite you to read the book, and reflect upon truth and practice simple ways of living. You've to align with Nature to be able to listen to the unique calls to heal your self. Let's ponder a little deeper in to your system and the Nature's design.

From Illness to Wellness!!!

Dedication

To my beloved Guru, Enlightened master, Maharishi Vethathiri, who is an eternal love! The one who has helped many scientistists in realization of truth.

Thank you. Without your support, I would have never achieved my dream.

From Illness to Wellness!!!

Note from the Author

My dear Brothers & Sisters,
                    Today, the World is astound with the etymology of diseases. It is increasing despite the technological advancements. Our human endeavor has reached the shores of Mars and Venus, whilst the plight of human beings in the planet, Earth is nearing an extinction.

Today. The World is haunted by the commoditized heathcare services which has no real intention of "healing" anyone, instead it is acting like a propaganda of infusing fears in your minds. It is being politized. Our human species is suffering from all sorts of health ailments with no proper healing methods. There is a wide GAP in terms of understanding the ancient wisdom in the contemporary medicines. You'll need to think about the diseases..A couple of hundred years ago, human beings were a lot healthier. The laser technology, scanning methods have profound wisdom but it is not helping in the end.

The transplantations are successful as they claim. But the patient's ailment continues, despite a successful transplantation. Eventually, at some point brain can be transplanted. But what will be the use of a vegetating live being. I would like to understand the real intent of the medicines, and technology.

From Illness to Wellness!!!

Unless it touches the lives of every human being to lead a healthy, and prosperous life...There is a lack of a holistic approach. I feel there is something lacking in the system, or perhaps a holistic method or application combining the ancient wisdom is lacking. You may call it as X, Y. Z disease, unless you're able to control the epidemic, the lists will increase in the future. The human species is slowly becoming the most endangered species today.

Friends, Today I'd like to invite you to think about the future & your children. A little glimpse of the healing techniques to let the Nature heal you. The profound Eastern wisdom of over five thousands years of wisdom to teach your children in simple ways of living in unison with the Nature.

I believe it is time for the medical science to comprehend the facts of ancient wisdom to be able to learn with the intuition provided by the ancient saints. They have lead a healthy life of over hundred years life span. Your forefathers were a lot healthier than you're now. This is leading me to believe technology has not really solved the problem, instead it is complicating your life more than ever in the commercialized world of "healthcare" services.
I request each of you to question the medicines prescribed and think about profound healing. Nature is providing you with symptoms to wake you up in the form of pains...If you take pain killer repeatedly, **you'll be painless in the end – leaving you DEAD!!!**

From Illness to Wellness!!!

Contents

Prologue 8
2025- World Health Organization (WHO) 8
The Healing Tree 10
Dealing with Illness 11
Rule # 1 – Know your Anatomy 18
Principles of Vedic Healing 24
Deficient Quantity/Quality of nutrients (Stage-1 vs. Stage-2): 25
CANCER 29
Remedy for Diseases 32
Nutrient Deficiency 36
Prevailing Diseases 38
NATURE'S HEALING 54
LEARN HEALING THERAPY METHOD 57
FOUR MAIN FACTORS OF DISEASES 58
INCREDIBLE FOUR DEFENSE MECHANISM 60
CHILD Birth Deficiencies 64
Vedic Healing 66
EYE SIGHT DEFECTS 67
KIDNEY Diseases 67
FIVE ATTRIBUTES OF WELLNESS 69
LIVER DISEASES 72
LUNG DISEASES 72
INFECTIONS 75
INFECTIONS IN KIDNEY 75
DIABETES 77
Rule # 5 – Discover simple ways of living 83
Tumor in Uterus 85
Appendicites 86
Thyroid 91
Vedic Secret Propounded 98

From Illness to Wellness!!!

Transformation of Taste 99
What happens to the food you eat? 99
YOU CAN CURE BP by SALT INTAKE 104
YOU CAN CURE DIABETES by SUGAR INTAKE 105
"SPICE" TASTE TREATMENT 107
"BITTER" Tatste Treatment 108
Process of Digestion 112
Vedic Rules of Eating Food 114
ADDICTIONS TO FOOD 134
Vedic Methods of Water Purification 135
AIR 138
Process of Breathing 139
EPILOGUE 156

From Illness to Wellness!!!

Prologue

2025- World Health Organization (WHO)

"A loud announcement in the 'WHO' auditorium filled with Scientists, Microbilogists, Doctors, celebrities and hollywood actors....

Dr.Sheela, the Director of WHO services analyzed achievements of renowned Doctors across the World. She finally called out the name loudly...The **'WHO'** services AWARD of the year **2025** goes to Dr.Guru, founder of the **'Vedic Healing Methods'** NGO (non-Governmental Organization) in India & the United States. Mr. Guru is a pioneer in healing millions of chronic illness to wellness. His holistic healing method is broadcasted across the World, with millions of followers.

Dr.Sheela explained about the profound vedic healing methods that has helped thousands of students all over the World cheering him in the workshop presentations. Above all, it is offered free of cost as a human birth right to surive healthy.

"May I request Dr.Guru to come on-stage please to receive the **'2025-WHO AWARD'** for the humanitarian services. Dr. has helped millions of students all over the World by conducting thousands of worshops". It has helped over a million viewers watching his programme through WHO broadcasts, podcasts and online meetings. These workshops have helped them get over diseases, it has saved them

From Illness to Wellness!!!

from the cronic illness. A countless have transformed themselves into a healthy & properous life.

"I would like to introduce Guru...who has been instrumental in helping students in every corner of the World with the '**Illness to Wellness**' program with simple and profound ways of living in helping them lead a healthy & prosperous life."

"**Ladies and Gentlemen**, Put your hands together for the gentlemen Guru. Today, the World is paranoid with the list of 'false' diseases and there is a little hope to the mankind. The list of diseases have increased. The rapid increase in the wellness center's have made you feel like patients and survivors of chronic illness, forming the list of celeberites."

Guru walks up to the stage to accept the award with flashing lights, photographers and press reporters applauding his tremendous feat of success! with the flashing cameras, Guru's thoughts were back to a few decades earlier....reminiscent in his memories of his mentor. Dr.Raj for his profound wisdom.

From Illness to Wellness!!!

The Healing Tree

Rule # 7 – Prevention is better than Cure

Rule # 6 – Healing Methods

Rule # 5 – Discover simple ways Of Living

Rule # 4 – Awareness about the Diseases

Rule # 3 – Transitional Therapy to Uproot your belief

Rule # 2 – Principles of Vedic Healing

Rule # 1 – Know your Anatomy (Body, Mind & Spirit)

The above **Healing** tree portrays the rules of healthy living, as you progress in each of these steps, you'll be able to achieve healthy life & success.

From Illness to Wellness!!!

1

Dealing with Illness

2000 – Bangalore Rehabilitation Center
Mr. Guru in his early 20's was working in T&L in North India. It was due to excessive stress & long hours at work, he had a sudden nervous break-down, he fell down unconscious. The ambulance carried him to the rehabilitation center to diagnose his condition. He was in a critical condition with a dropping pulse rate. The next morning he woke up in Dr.Raj's Medical center, finding a Dr. examining his condition.

"You'll be al right. Just get some rest." As Dr. flashes his report.

Guru worked as a Civil Engineer in the Toubro & Larson (T&L), one of the larget construction company in India. A few months later Guru relocated to South Chennai, where he visited Dr.Raj's medical center in South Chennai...Guru is asking Raj if he could help him heal the condition.

"Dr.Can you help my condition?"

"I just checked your scan results, blood tests, everything is absolutely fine."

From Illness to Wellness!!!

Dr. interrupts….

Is that you? Guru from Mumbai….!
"Dr. Yes. I am Guru from Mumbai. You had treated me in the Mumbai Medical center…"
"Oh boy!!! I rememeber. I treated you in the Mumbai Medical center every month. You were very critical! "

"I've heard about your Vedic Healing sessions…broadcasted last Friday in the WHO!"
"Oh, You're talking about the 'Illness to Wellness program broadcasted lastnight'…Isn't?"

"Yes. Dr!"

"Yup. That was a grand success in the WHO, broadcasted over fifty countries in the World. I've been getting calls from different Regions to conduct workshops frequently. Unfortunately, I have less bandwidth and team to support a large Global programme…"

"Well. That's is exactly why I am here Dr." as Guru responded.
"I'll need your help!!!!"

"Guru. Sure, I can help you. You'll need to go through the fourteen sessions as part of the workshops to understand the **'Vedic Healing techniques'**"

"Dr. interrupts. I would like basic tests & details of your ailment prior to the workshops. You've been going through regular headache, constipation etc.. for years since your

From Illness to Wellness!!!

childhood. Oh my GOD, none of these Doctors could help you! It's a pity my dear friend!!!! as the Dr. emphathizes him."

"So What happened to you!"
"Dr. I don't know…This is happening since my childhood. I was working for T&L as a Sr.Architect. I was paid very highly, regarded as highest paid by Indian standards,…One fine day, I just quit the job due to my deteoriating health."

"I boarded the train from Mumbai, reached Bangalore. I fell down at the bus station in Bangalore, and remained unconscious for a few days..I regained myself after a week and came back to my hometown..here I am!"

"'I see…' as Dr. flipping was through the case history!"
"OK Dr. Please meet me with the ECG report & the case history details of your condition next week for the workshops."

"I suggest you continue with the medications until the workshops. Will discuss further by next week.."
"Good that all these results are negative!"

The following week:
"Well. Mr. Guru, that is certainly a progress.
With the documents, evidence of Guru's ECG analysis and brain scan test results." Now, it is late in the evening. Doctor was ready to leave the office carrying all his patients profile to home.

"Bye". Guru started whispering with a sigh of relief.

From Illness to Wellness!!!

Dr. Raj was surveying Guru's profile to find the recent historical records; he flipped through individual records and he stumbled on this one for Mr. Guru's case study in specific:

" I fell down unconscious twice, and it has been happening since my childhood...with frequent migraine, sleepless disorders and experiences of trauma."

Dr.Raj realized the conditioning was an **mental and physical** as highlighted in the journal of medicine. Perhaps it was not properly diagnosed by the medical community as he thought to himself, reading through the rest of the patient's case study. He had immense wisdom of healing techniques of the East combined with modern science.

Often, he treated patients with a holistic view and his research on diseases was not just external, as it is mostly internal due to lack of understanding Nature's subtle messages. Dr.Raj was not just a clinician, but also a practitioner of ancient Pranic healing techniques & Nature's healing methods, with extensive knowledge in the Eastern Philosphy.

Dr. continues...

"Guru, your condition is not critical, however you'll need to go through the therapy sessions planned. In fact, I'd call it an alternate approach to healing to help you transform your life from illness to welless."

From Illness to Wellness!!!

Guru left the clinic with a sigh of relief, and regained hope after several years of desparate attempts to cure his ailments through the medications, none of which had helped him.

"Yes. It does. But, the techniques that I am going to teach you is not physical, it is mental. It will help you change your perceptions and alter your priorities to suceed."

"Thanks Dr." as Guru responded like a kid back to school to learn the techniques.

"Let's start with the basic analysis. Do you understand the anatomy?"
"Do you observe how negligent you are by taking temporary medications, resulting in major illness?"

"Yes Dr. I take a lot of aspirins!"
"That's the starting point. A head ache could be Nature's subtle message to you about stress or something else. If you take aspirin, you just suppress all these messages!"

"Dr.What will the result then?"
"The result will be a disaster. A long term consequence of dieseases could possibly cause diseases such as Cancer."

"Uh ....I haven't thought about that!"
"Ok. Let me tell you something..."

Look at this formula:

From Illness to Wellness!!!

Health Quotient (HQ) = KYA+PVH+TT............(1)
1. Know your Anatomy (KYA)
2. Principles of Vedic Healing (PVH) &
3. Transitional Therapy (TT)

Wellness Quotient (RQ) =
AAD+DWL+HTS+PBC...............................(2)
1. Awareness about the Dieseases (AAD)
2. Discover simple ways of living (DWL)
3. Heal thy self (HTS)
4. Prevention is better than cure (PBC)

These are simple acronymns to memorize. It will help you suceed as you progress in the workshops.
Ok. In first three topics, you'll be analyzing your health. I'll teach you how to manage your health to get over your diseases, which is the formula for the Health Quotient (HQ)'
"Great. Thanks Dr."

In the last four topics, you'll know about the healing methods, and your organic unit with Nautre, which is the formula for the Wellness Quotient (RQ).

"Interesting."

"Fasten your seat belts on…to learn something very exciting, which will change your life forever. You will need to practice these exercises discussed post the session, and contemplate deeply to understand the profound techniques. I've conducted these sessions all over the World to benefit over millions of students, & entrepreneurs to tranform their illness to welleness."

From Illness to Wellness!!!

You'll be transformed to a great leader by the end of the 14th Session. There is Q&A planned at the end of every session to answer all queries that you may have.

"Thanks Dr." as Guru is prepared to learn once again, back to school. The real school of Altruism!!!

*

A few years later, GURU master's these healing techniques and conducts workshops Worldwide !!!

***

From Illness to Wellness!!!

Day 1 - Session # 1: Know your Anatomy (**KYA**)

Rule # 1 – Know your Anatomy

Siddhas of India have identified three layers of body, which are:

1. **Physical Body** – Physical body is made up of cells,
2. **Astral Body** – Astral body is made up of life force (energy) particles &
3. **Causal Body** – Causal body is the magentic body or Atma.

You're organically connected with the mother. Nature. THE ABOVE three layers shouldn't be disturbed.

Human Physiology

You often forget the holistic view of your body, mind & spirit. Would you smoke a Cigar, if you are aware of the respiratory system....or perhaps you would refrain from alcohol if you know the harmful effects? And how much damage you bring in to the gift that you have been endowed with by Mother Nature....Nature has planned it meticulously and it took millions of years to arrive at

From Illness to Wellness!!!

human anatomy far far superior from the animals in terms of organs, and senses to perceive transformation of magnetism. Is it not a wonder as you ponder, to comprehend the grace, intellect and beauty of the Mother Nature? Let's explore some important points of your anatomy...

Everyone will agree functions of brain...hence there is no need to explain in greater detail which is part of the nervous system and controls everything in your body, let us analyze all other functions in layman terms... the sensory perceptions of touch, smell, taste are received by brain. Heart is the center of blood circulation for oxygenating blood, by pumping blood to all parts of your body & Lungs are the center of air circulation for oxygen exchange in your body.   .

The kidneys are a part of the endocrine system. These organs provide necessary filtration of metabolic waste in tissue cells. The stomach and Intestines. .which holds food as you all know and sends it to intestines for digestion and absorption. The pancreas and gallbladder provides enzymes to breakdown the stomach contents. The metabolic waste is sent down the colon, and removed during bowel moments.

Hence, I would like to emphasize on level of the awareness on how much you owe to Nature itself for the beautiful system, and more and more you contemplate on nervous system and your organ functions and activities...remember it is not something which has happened by overnight... The ultimate truth has planned your body, mind and soul

From Illness to Wellness!!!

for designing you, and above all it loves you to the core.

Do you agree 'Love is that which hold incessantly'. He would never let you suffer. All sufferings are man-made and fake as you fail to comprehend Truth and its Cause and Effects. All conflicts can be resolved intellectually; Perhaps GOD need not be disturbed as you have been gifted with Mind to analyze. If you find it difficult to meditate initially, you should start preparing your body in simple Yoga exercises including breathing, and follow for some time…eventually it will lead to meditation.

Your Mind acts in psychic extension of consciousness in feeling, Thus it functions as this: need, sensation, zeal, action, result, enjoyment, experience, research, realization and conclusion as described as "Mind" There are three needs. Hunger, climatic sensation and excretion of waste from your body. And the countless energy particles are thrown out of your body continuously due to the rotation of the Earth, and you feel hunger for refilling.

Arabian Proverb for you to ponder!
"The one who has hope has everything;
The one who has health has hope!"

From Illness to Wellness!!!

CELL PHYSIOLOGY

The cells are the building blocks of your body. Let us imagine cell like a house, and the blood stream as a road. You are flying in a helicopter, an aerial view of houses and roads. Once the home (cell) opens it door to extract sugar (glucose) from the blood.

Mitochondria is like a car in the house, which will need "fuel" to run. The fuel is 'sugar' that has been extracted a while ago from the blood. Now, your car will need air to burn the fuel. Hence, your cells will extract Oxygen from blood. Now, imagine countless millions of cells performing the above action of extracting sugar from the blood and exchange Oxygen to do some work through Mitochondria.

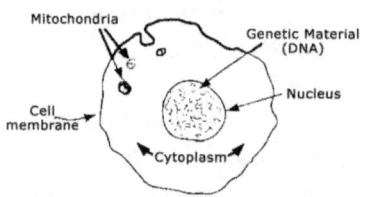

SNO	Constituents	Function
1	The Nucleus	Center. Site of DNA, enclosed by a membrane
2	Mitochondria	Extract energy from FOOD FUEL
3	Anaerobic Metabolism	Glycolysis is anaerobic-carried out in cytosol
4	Aerobic Metabolism	Combines with Coenzyme A loosing a CO_2 and becoming Acetyl Coenzyme A (2 C fragment)
5	THE CYTOSKELETON	Microtubules
6	DNA/RNA	Genetic strands

From Illness to Wellness!!!

What do you observe from the above phenomena?

The cell function is same from the cells in your hair to the toes, however the functions will vary depending on the organs functions. Once the fuel is burnt and the work is done, the residue goes out as an exhaust right in your car. In a similar terms, your cells will perform its function by burning sugar, and the residue is Urea. Your cell will turn this residue (Urea) back into the blood stream. Your cell has already used the Oxygen, once work is done it turns into residue as Carbondioxide. It is thrown out of cell (home) to the blood stream (road). Your cell (home) will extract necessary nutrient from blood and it varies depending on the needs and work done every second. Each cell has its own intelligence, and it rejuvenates constantly.

Your body is made up of "Pancha Boothas". Each of your organ is connected to it.

SNO	ELEMENT	ORGANS
1	LAND	Bones, Muscles
2.	WATER	Blood, Water
3.	FIRE	Body Temperature. Oxygen in Body
4.	AIR	Air, Lungs
5.	Space	Atma

End of Session # 1.

From Illness to Wellness!!!

Questions to Ponder?
1. A real medicine is to heal you completely. Ask yourself if your BP/DIABETES etc. medications have increased or reduced over a period of time?
2. Have you increased or reduced the dosage of medications?
3. Did you completely RECOVER from the illness?
4. If your sickness is cured or repeating?

If the answer is no, then it is imperative that your ailments are not cured completely, A holistic healing method is required. There is a need to reinvent the methods of ancient healing practices of India. These Siddha's had lived longer and healthier for centuries. There seems to be missing intelligence of siddhic tradition. Let us try to analyze the basics of human physiology, organ functions and cell structure etc. I insist Doctors, Microbiologists and Scientists to realize the values of the ancient healing methods for a holistic treatment.

***

From Illness to Wellness!!!

2

Principles of Vedic Healing

Now, let us analye the basic differences in the way allopathy is treating patients with the ancient healing methods. Our ancient healing methods involve treating your diseases at the root, meaning to give you required organic cure to boost the immunity in 'blood'.

You'll be healed by following simple & profoud ways of living thus governing your regular FOOD quantity & quality, REST, WORK, sexual vital fluid & Thoughts. Each of it should be within limits as per the LAWS of NATURE. The above principle of treating it at the root is identifying the nutrients deficiencies in bloood to boost the natural immune system. This holistic treatment will be a paradigm shift in the history of medical journal by combining the best practices of siddhic healing methods.

The fundamental theory in medical journal is not treating diseases at the root. Adding to that the commoditized healthcare have changed the real motto of healing vs. temporary relief. I am afraid the real intent has been lost.

From Illness to Wellness!!!

The vedic healing method propounds methods to treat diseases at the root in blood. The deficiencies in blood is analyzed based on symptoms and healed with natural cure with herbs and food that will boost the defence mechanism in blood.

Deficient Quantity/Quality of nutrients (Stage-1 vs. Stage-2):

There are two stages in diseases. First it will start with the Stage-1 as deficiency of "quality" a main nutrient in blood such as calcium, sodium etc. The second Stage-2 is the deficiency of more than one nutrient quantiy in blood. In healing, we heal with remedy in Step-1 itself. The consequence of a disease will be higher with its impact to the Organs, depending on the stage-1 or stage-2 & stage-3 is chronic illness.

In Stage-1, after you take necessary medications as prescribed by the Doctors. You'd complain there is lack of quanity of Calcium, Sodium, Magnesium, Iodine etc. Instead of healing at this Stage-1. Your Doctors will prescribe medicines that will push you to Stage-2, which means the medications will make other nutrients deficient in blood below the critical level. Thus, you'll become completely DEFICIENT of core NUTRIENTS in BLOOD. This is what your Allopathy is capable of doing to each of you! Perhaps, the stage-3 becomes chronic illness, resulting in ORGAN failures. We will discuss simple methods to improve the quality & quantity NUTRIENTS in blood through simple ways of vedic methods of living.

From Illness to Wellness!!!

Reasons for the Deficient Quantity of Blood (Heamogobin, Anemic- Stage-3)

This is termed as stage-3 DISEASE with the reduced quantity of blood. Each of you will have a specific required quantity of blood, depending on **AGE, HEIGHT & WEIGHT. Let's explore the reasons.**
The bone marrow is responsible for rejuvenating the new blood cells based on the quality of blood available. When the quality reduces, it will lose its ability to produce new blood cells, resulting in a deficient quality of blood. I'll teach you the method to maintain good quality of blood to avoid chronic illness.

Mind Power

Your mind is wave is linked to the physical body. A disturbed MIND will cause all sorts of ailments. There is a close relation between the BODY, MIND as discussed. If you're SICK, BODY will impact MIND as you cannot think properly. Your emotions will impact the glands. If your BODY is at discomfort, MIND cannot rest in peace & vice versa.

The impact will be both in MIND, and BODY. If your MIND power is diluted, you'll be prone to the diseases. If you're able to enhance your MIND POWER, you'll have the inbuilt healing system supporting your physiology for a quick recovery. Your depressions will drain the MIND POWER, causing ailments in the physiology. In summary, both are interlinked. You should try to remain silent to improve your MIND POWER by the way of meditation and introspective analysis to eliminate deppressions. This will boost your IMMUNE levels.

From Illness to Wellness!!!

Your MIND POWER is proportionate to the Quantity & Quality of the Sexual vital fluid. If your sexual vital fluid is liquidated through excessive behavior, it will lead to chronic illness as your BODY will lose its IMMUNITY.
End of Session # 2.

Day 2 – Session # 3: Let's analyze few diseases.
After a couple of phenomenal sessions, Guru was even more enthusiastic to learn the art of transformation. We have received some good news from the Moon TV channel to broadcast our 'Healing' methods. "That's a real good news;" as Guru said, tasting the hot filter coffee.

"Thambi , Kapi nanna Erukkuda." (coffee is good!)

"Anna. Nanri. Edhu filter coffee."
"Ok. Let's get back to the topics. Can you swith on the projector?"

"You've passed the first two sessions, now the third one is really simple."
"What is it Dr."

Identifying the diseases....

Disruption in the Cell Intelligent System
Your CELL intelligence will work perfectly fine without any intervention, however when you spoil your senses by excessive usage..You'll end up in forming a trend of draining bio-magnetism in the

From Illness to Wellness!!!

respective Organs. As a result, your rate of conversion in the respective Organ is much higher than the normal usage of the sense Organs. Your sense ORGANSs will deviate with upper limits of conversion of bio-magnetism unit/sec, thus enforcing cells to increase its whirling motion. These cells will lose its polarity without following the cell consciousenss and the instructions within due to the lost polarity. It will try to balance by speeding up its whirling motion. When the sense organs accelerate its usage. Cells will tend to whirl much faster than usual and the conversion rate is higher. These sense organs are organically linked to the whole physiology, thus impacting the internal organs as well. Perhaps, you've done something unknowingly to mess up with the natural cell intelligence that orders for renewal of RBC and WBC's. This in turn will activate required killer proteins to succeed against diseases.

However, in this case if you are unable to produce required "killer" protein, due to the non-renewed WBC's. and the cells will eventually die. This is cancer. You've to rebuild the intelligence. There is no way you can cure by doing multiple sessions of Heamotherapy, which will not help in the longer run. It will suppress the count of WBC's without rebuilding the intelligence to renew it automatically. Do you see my point! Its like a car engine oil quality has degrated. You're trying to fix everything else except supplying a good quality oil. The same analogy here is blood. If you improve the quality of blood..everything else will be healed.

From Illness to Wellness!!!

Defense Mechanism

Whenever there is a germ entering your blood, the first step will be your Organs, which will form a committee such as Thymus, Liver, WBC, Bone Marrow & Kidney to research about the germs, create a solution to kill the germs with the help of a "Killer" Protein from blood itself. However, if the sexual vital fluid is liquidated then the main nutrients in blood will not be available to prepare necessary killer "PROTEINS" as part of the DEFENCE mechanism. This would result in the DEFENCE mechanism failing to protect you. IT is mainly due to the liquidated sexual vital fluid, which cannot support your "Killer" Proteins with vitality to DEFENCE against the diseases. End result, your DISEASE will triumph. The LOST ability OF THE cell consciousness to resist DISEASES or rquired IMMUNE to DEFEND DISEASES is "AIDS (Acquired Immune Deficiency Syndrome)".

Perhaps you've altered the DEFENSE mechanism so much through the excessive sexual behavior causing misaligned cellular polarity. Thus, your blood cells have lost the ability to produce Killer proteins to DEFEND. Your excessive sexual behavior result in liquidated 'sexual vital fluid', which is the source of Prana shakthi within your body. Thus leaving you prone to diseases.

CANCER

For example. Cancer is a disease due to the lost cell intelligence. In your cell physiology, WBC rejuvenates itself every 13 days, RBC rejuvenates itself in every

From Illness to Wellness!!!

120 days, and Liver rejuvenates every year, intestines will do every 36 hours so on and so forth. If your Organs lose the ability to rejuvenate itself as indicated above will result in a disease called **CANCER.** Let's say if your WBC's will need to rejuvenate every 13 DAYS, Now it has lost its ability and rejuvenates later in 330 DAYS instead of 13 DAYS. During that time of rejuvenation the count of WBC's will vary significantly lower, say for example < 4,500, wherein the normal count should be 4,500 to 11,500. This is called **BLOOD CANCER.** On the contrary if WBC rejuvenates every 13 minutes instead of 13 days. This would result in the blood CANCER? The **"HEAMOTHERAPY"** treatments that is prescribed will increase/reduce the WBC. This will not solve the problem of the "Cell consciouses" which is causing the timing change in the rate of rejuvenating your body cells. Only the cell conscoiusness will need to be corrected, not the WBC's in the blood.

If the cells in the BONE fail to rejuvenate on-time, it would result in **BONE CANCER.** In summary the rapid rejuvenation or the delayed rejuvenation of the cells will result in CANCER. In either case it is chronic and there are no treatments available except **for the "HEAMOTHERAPY" as discussed above. If it fails to rejuvenate at ORGAN level is termed as ORGAN CANCER.**

ONE of the reason for the **LOST INTELLIGENCE to** rejuvenate is due to the Stage-1–4 as discussed above. The allopathy medications taken in over a period of time has defied the Natural alert mechanism,

From Illness to Wellness!!!

eventually your CELLS would give up in trying to rejuvenate as you've altered the Nature's intrinsic program. It is like you've decoded the IBM or MS software & the application failed to execute. You update the patches without a proper debug analysis, what will happen next? Your application will crash eventually with a point of no-return. This is exactly what is happening. Through the excessive medicines you've altered the Nature's inherent potential to rejuvenate itself!!! You've messed up with the Nature's program.

Remember, Lost cell intelligence (liquidated vital energy) in the system to rejuvenate the CELLS is CANCER. Above all, our scriptures have indicated sensual enjoyment in moderation. If the excesss limits are reached, then it will lead to misalignment of cell structure, & polarity causing all sorts of ailments. Moreso, these chronic diseases don't kill a patient overnight. It is a process which will take years, however Doctors response by stating it to the patients, would kill them in months due to the deppressions adding to the physical ailments. The good news is that you will be HEALED if you BELIEVE in Nature's cure. THE VEDIC HEALING WILL PROVIDE YOU WITH PROFOUD WAYS TO HEAL YOURSELF, WHICH NO MEDICINES CAN CURE.

These deficiencies can be healed by the following Q2Mel Formula factors:

From Illness to Wellness!!!

Remedy for Diseases

SNO	FIVE MAIN FACTORS OF DISEASES	REMEDY
1.	Quantity of blood	Eat Good food and digest it completely by following simple methods
2.	Quality of blood including main constituents	Enhance quality of blood through food with required intake of calcium, sodium, carbohydrates etc.
3.	Mind Energy	Improve through MEDITATION/Yoga Sadhana to restore energy
4.	**Cell Intelligence - Quality/Quantity Life Force or** The ability to respond which is the Cell's Intelligent system.	You should maintain quality & quantity of Sexual Vital Fluid with intercourse in moderation with disturbing the cellular polarity & its inherent intelligence to solve

We will discuss REMEDY steps as we progress in greater details. Let's call it as **"Q2MeL"** (pronounce it as Q-Square-Mel).

End of Session # 3

From Illness to Wellness!!!

Day 3 – Session # 4: Transtional Therapy
Rule # 3 Transitional Therapy to Uproot your view of Diseases

Did you analyze the way you perceive diseases?

HDL. LDL Cholesterol

FAT

HDL

LDL Once again we have Good Cholesterol (HDL) vs. Bad Cholesterol (LDL) in blood. A good cholesterol is properly digested food and the bad is due to improper digestion of food with residue fat. "HDL" refers to the High Density Lipo protein & LDL refers to the Low density lipo protein. A proper digestion of food will lead to good cholesterol and vice versa. LDL or bad cholestrol would eventually form fat tumors in blood. These LDL will start blocking the blood vessels.

These blood vessles are blocked due to the increasing no. of fat tumors formed by "LDL" or BAD cholesterol, this would result in a high Blood Pressure. (BP). Whicever Organ receiving this bad cholesterol will be impacted. Your BILE fluid secreted will segreate BAD cholestrol and deposit in the GALL BLADDER. The fluid from harmone will help in digestion, however due to the BAD cholestrol it will

From Illness to Wellness!!!

not secrete required quality of fluids to support in digestion. As a result the blood vessels to the heart will be choked due to excess desposites in the vessel, casuing heart attack.

Hence, you'll need to understand the fact that it is due to the improper digestion of food, leading to the "BAD" cholesterol, resulting in heart attacks. Now, ask a question. Who is the cause? You're the culprit for not eating quality food. While we thank the medical World for the 'ANGIOGRAM' method to deblock the congestion, a procedure used for removing the bad cholesterol. **How insane is to completely avoid food without cholesterol?** Cholesterol is one of the main ingredient required for cell functions. If you deny intake of any food with cholesterol, this will lead to a major disaster.

 "Good Cholesterol is good for your cells."

Your cells are clinging to each other like bricks in houses. And GOOD cholesterol is like cement helping in clinging to each. It is good cholesterol that helps in patching cells together. Hence, you should change the way you eat food to digest completely to be able to convert it to good cholesterol.

DID YOU KNOW...BILE fluid is secreted by the LIVER and stored in the GALL BLADDER for absorption of fat. This fluid is essental for digestion. The oily fat on the surface of skin is essential to protect you from the SKIN diseases.

From Illness to Wellness!!!

The essense in healing method is to teach you methods to eat food that will convert it to good cholesterol. I'll teach you a simple technique of how to eat food to convert to good cholesterol. I'd say **"Cocunut"** is the best food in the WORLD, Hence in ancient Hinduism "COCUNUT" had a place in every offering to GOD. It indicates the importance of the ancient Wisdom. One of the profound wisdom is that a simple healing from Cocunut milk, in ancient days if no medicine works for a patient, as a last resort they tried cocunut milk and it worked in most of the intances to heal the diseased. This is one of the profound method followed in ancient days!

I've observed the youngsters are alergic to "Oily" foods, especially mostly women who are conscious about the weight loss. Perhaps this remains the only global rule at the expense of lost health in torturing the body in the name of DIET. DIET is a four letter word that women should be carefully assess to avoid mal-nutrition!!!

There is no need to avoid "OILY" food. You'll need OIL with fat, hence do not go by the advertisements of "OIL" with fat removed. The purpose is to extract good fat from OIL to help your cells. "**SESAME** (a.k.a YELLU in tamil)" OIL is the best.
If you practice good eating habits, and the oil intake as required quanity will eventually drive away all BAD cholesterol.

From Illness to Wellness!!!

Nutrient Deficiency

We have observed diseases are due to the quality of blood deteriating. Let's analyze the specifics of why it is deficient in few nutrients? If your blood is deficient of SUGAR, then the disease is called DIABETES. Let's review the table below:

NO	Deficiencies in Blood	Disease
1	Deficiency in SUGAR LEVEL	DIABETES
2	Deficiency in Calcium level	Bone diseases
3	Deficincy in Calcium, Sodium & Iodine etc.	Thyroid
4	Deficiency in Vitamin A	Eye Sight & many other diseases
5	Deficiency in Vitamin D	Arthoritics, Joints & many more
6	Deficiency in Vitamin B	Skin diseases
7	Deficiency in Vitamin K	Ability to Blood Clot will not be possible.

If you've eye sight problems, you should try & resolve Vitamin A deficiencies to cure yourself with simple eye exercies such as candle light gazing. There is no point in treating EYE alone in isolation or surgery is not a remedy. In similar terms deficiencies in Vitamin D would cause Arthoritics, there is no point in treating your nees in isolation. You'll need to understand the paradigm shift in treating all your diseases by identifying deficiences in blood. This is

From Illness to Wellness!!!

the best method & and a holistic view of healing your body.

A simple analogy. If you observe a house on fire, with all windows closed except for one window open. You'll observe gush smoke coming out of the window. Would you identify fire in a single room or the entire building. You'd comprehend the fire is on the building and the room is severly impacted. Your whole cell physiology is impacted by the deficiency, however a specific organ that is weaker is impacted first. Instead of treating it organically, if you just treating the Organs will not help.

You've mastered the first three rules of The Illness toWellness;

1. Identify your '**ANATOMY**' (IYA);
2. Principles of Vedic Healing (AT);
3. Transitional THERAPY (TT);

End of Session # 4.

From Illness to Wellness!!!

3

Prevailing Diseases

Day 4 – Session # 5: Awareness about the Diseases
The fifth session was ecstatic as Guru started enjoying every moment...
"Guru, We will discuss the various facets of diseases & reasons a little more deeply, and the CAUSE. You have realized the essence of "**PAIN**" and the unfolding "**SICKNESS**"."

You'll need to analyze the factors causing diseases.
Rule # 4 Awareness about the Diseases
"Guru..Could you write about your ailments on the board please"
"SURE" as he walks to the board to write:

FEVER   SINUS
HEADACHE   TUBERCLOSIS
DYSENTRY   RUNNING NOSE
ASTHMA   Blood Pressure

Perhaps. I'd rephrase. These are symptoms of your body's alert system. It is going through the process of healing. You'll need to change your ideology about diseases.

Well. Let's discuss.
The only investment that I will need from you is

From Illness to Wellness!!!

patience to listen to your body. This will heal you totally! It's your mind which has complicated everything, Nature has profound wisdom. You've to believe in mother. Nature, she will heal you through the discourses. There is no scientific evidence required as I am going to explain you how the glands are activated while you're listening through the heart and spirit. It's a profound method from the ancient Vedic scriptures in India.

You should practice listening to the inner system. Nature has created you with absolute pattern, precision and regularity meaning every cell in the body has a set of tasks to perform which transforms eventually into Organ functions. It's a perfect system and you interfere into each of its function, resulting in diseases. An interruption in the natural rhythm is perceived as a disease.

What is a DISEASE?

A disease is a disturbance in the cellular structure. It originates from blood and impacts an organ if not healed properly. The ancient vedic healing method will help you cure the internal diseases, such as diabetes, asthma, BP, Sinus, Cancer, hair fall, skin diseases, head-ache, eye sight, glaucoma, running nose, TB, few heart diseases, Pneumonia, kidney failure, Digestive problems, sexual disorders, women menstrual problems, slip disc etc. The vedic (siddha) treatment is intended for most of the internal diseases.

From Illness to Wellness!!!

You don't need to fear any germs, virus or bacteria, as a matter of fact you've been living in and around millions of organisms in the atmosphere. If you have headache, DO NOT take aspirins as a short remedy. Relax and diagnose yourself for the root causes of stress or something else. If you take aspirin you're perhaps numbing down the neurons to temporarily halt the Nature's alert mechanism. It will not help in anyways as the sickness is not cured or diagnosed correctly. Just throw away ASPIRINS, PAIN KILLERS & sleeping pills etc. They are of no use to heal the condition. All sleeping pills are dangerous, perhaps it can be a one-time usage for a specific purpose but definetly not on a regular basis.

It has to be a natural method to heal your condition. Let's see step by step process how your diseases start, perhaps how negligent you're to the bio-natural alert system. First of all, you'll need to understand the health chart. Your health ailments start in steps. No one will become diseased over-night. It is a process and it takes time. If you are aware, all you need to do is to let the DIVINE heal you. The following flow chart indicate the diseases progressing starting from respiratory system to skin with symptoms in every stages. You can treat these diseases at the root.

From Illness to Wellness!!!

Progressing Diseases

STEP 1 – Respiratory System. This is the beginning stage of any disease.
STEP 2 – Digestive System. This is the next stage of the diseases
STEP 3 – SKIN

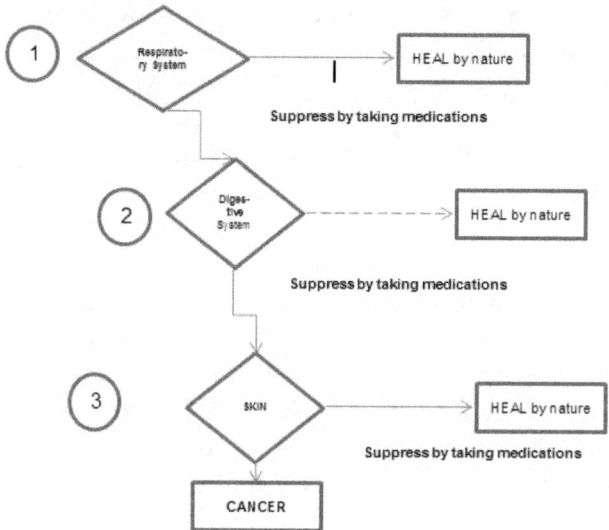

DID YOU SEE MY POINT? The beginning of any diseases is due to suppression of the specific natural alarm. Like suppressing your sneeze through the medications, or fever. Perhaps your allopathy medicines didn't go to the roots of the diseases, instead you've treated by temporarliy halting the alert mechanism. A simple analogy is like a pressure cooker releasing its pressure through the gasket valve. If you let go, your food is cooked properly boiled and turn it off once done. If you interrupt by forcing the pressure, it will burn the food isn't?

From Illness to Wellness!!!

It's a simple release mechanism to let the pressure go. In a similar analogy, a simple and profound method proposed by Nature is to alert you using the glands that will secret as appropriately to switch on the alert system. It happenes from a simple sneeze to the large diseases. You should NOT supess it through immediate medications. A disease is nothing but the net sum of your suppressions. Let us explore how it happnes in this process, and how you've been ignoring Nature's alert system. A simple and profound breathing pattern such as '**Kabala pathi**' can throw away infections in lungs through a pattern of breathing.

I hear your BODY saying:
"DO NOT MESS UP WITH ME.
IF YOU ARE GOOD. I'LL BE GOOD TO YOU."

Respiratory System

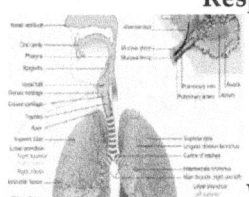

WHY DO YOU SNEEZE?

Your sneeze is due to the pollution in the lungs. It is a labyrinthine of coordination with your physiology. When the lungs are clogged with infections through air, these objects have to be thrown out of the body. The HI THYAMINE gland will be activated to perform this operation. Eventually, you'll sneeze twice or thrice depending on the quantity of the foreign object to be thrown out.

If you are trying to stop sneeze or perhaps use a balm to stop it, it will result in performing an anti-action

From Illness to Wellness!!!

within your own system. It will hinder the functions of the HI THYAMINE GLAND resulting in toxins in your body.

RUNNING NOSE

The ultimate DR. within you had activated the SNEEZE therapy to throw the foreign objects However, if it exceeds an alarmingly a high no, then the sneeze will fall back on a different option as it will not work if the lungs have accumulated pollution beyond a specified limits. It will initiate the 'RUNNING NOSE' GLAND to wash out the dirt deposited in the lungs. It is synonymous to a vacuum cleaner used in the house with liquid soap to mop the floor. Indeed, the irony is whenever you're affected with 'RUNNING NOse', which indicates Nature is providing an option to clean the lungs. If you stop by using antibiotics or perhaps inhaling the liquid will result in negative consequences. RUNNING NOSE is good. You should exhale to remove all the fluids in the nose which would remove infections in the body (germs).

SINUS/ASTHMA & TUBERCLOSIS

In the above analogy, if you avoid exhaling the fluids in the nose, then you're allowing the deposit of germs in to your lungs. As a result it will multiple almost more than tenfold. This is the root cause of **SINUS**. When your Dr. prescribes antibiotics to control fluids in nose, it will increase the headcount further in the lungs as deposits. And finally antibiotics will activate the gland to control the

From Illness to Wellness!!!

foreign objects. This activation will have negative conequences.

If you take medications for running nose, which indicates you're aggravating the condition resulting in diseases & your medications impact the IMMUNE system. I have personally experienced in my life as I was taking medications for running nose, apparently it had resulted in depositing in lungs turning as 'flum' in the chest, and severe caughing. An increased 'FLUM' (FLUIDS) in the chest with congestion in breathing turns to ASTHMA.

If the infections exceed a certain limit, it will block the passage of lungs, and trachea (wind pipe). As a result, the breathing is interrupted causing **'WHEEZING'**. This extended condition in your lungs with an increasing headcount of infections would result in Tuberclosis. Indeed, the irony is that Nature had indicated through SNEEZE, and then eventually through the second step process of **RUNNING NOSE**..If you further do not relent to it by exhaling the fluids…instead, you inhale and deposited the infections by temporarily halting the respective glands by using interim medications. Do you see my point of how Allopathic treatments work? It's like fixing your vehicle individually in the spare parts without proper diagnosis, resulting in one hundred and one different problems.

These medications will finally aggravate the situation, resulting in large deposits of foreign objects in your lungs, passage to the nose resulting in **'Tuberculosis'**

From Illness to Wellness!!!

and congestion through the nasal passage. A simple analogy is to take your vehicle to the nearest mechanic, where the real problem is with the oil filter. You were replacing everything else as adviced by the mechanic without proper diagnosis. After all the steps, you would still hear engine noise, now the mechanic says…you Engine condition has worsened and the only way out is to replacing it.

This is what your Doctors are doing through diagnosis. They do one hundred and one scanning at the organs and finally evaluate incorrectly with medicines that will aggravate the situation, resulting in surgery upto removal of organs. A disease is a result of your ignorance. Ignorance is not bliss in adults, as you're being taken for granted in allopathic treatments.

Digestive System

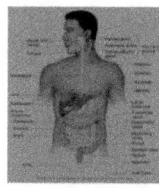 **PUKE**

When you had eaten a spoiled food. Your stomach organ has its consciousness to identify, segregate the good vs. bad food. If food is spoiled, it will try to throw it out. This is puking **'VOMITTING'** is good as it is a built in intelligence within your body to throw away excessive food or spoiled food within your body based on the consciousness with in your stomach organ. It has healed the condition. What you've done thoughtlessly by dumping some food

From Illness to Wellness!!!

into stomach has been thrown out by the Natural process in the form of vomiting. Indeed, this is Nature's cast to remove pollution from the internal system. Say for instance. If you take medications to stop 'vomiting'...remember, you're interrupting Nature's system. Hence, you end up depositing it back into the stomach. If you take medications to stop the vomiting sensations, which indicate you've forced your system to digest the "garbage" in your stomach, which was otherwise meant to be thrown out of the system.

You should thank Nature as it has designed a system to correct from your mistake. It is performing the corrective action to heal the system by itself. Hope you'll not interfere with the system anymore.

✓ I'd suggest taking lemon juice after you vomit completely. This will further cleanse the stomach and correct the digestive track, however please remember NOT to take lemon juice prior to vomiting to cleanse the intestines.

DIARRHEA

Your intestines are completely choked by now due to infections in stomach by way of food or air. Nature will activate the respective 'Dysentry' gland to throwing the digested junk food or perhaps an accumulated waste due to constipation. Indeed, this is part of Nature's design to cleanse your intestines by throwing out the stacked garbage in the system. While the whole WORLD is thinking loud in treating waste...and waste management. Nature has meticulously planned to treat your inner waste in the

From Illness to Wellness!!!

intestines by activating the 'Dysentry' GLAND to throw the garbage out of the system. In summary it is an intestine cleansing act casted by Nature.

You'll feel tired if you have passed out few times. You should take a) water b) glucose & c) salt to compensate the loss in your body. Once you recover from dysentery, try some light natural food before eating cooked or baked food. If you're trying to interrupt dysentery, or perhaps by taking medications to stop dysentery will result in diseases.

FEVER

Indeed you've violated the Natural laws by disrupting the flow in the first place. Without realizing its value, you've have interrupted the step 1 – medications to avoid running nose, step – 2 – your body has an electro-meter gland, that takes care of body temperature. It controls every Organ to maintain a body temperature of 98.4 degree Fahrenheit, regardless of wherever you stay. Hence, it is imperative to understand the Nature's design. Did you think why would your body run a very high temperature suddenly? Don't you think there is any reason to it?

Indeed, Nature is trying to throw the accumulated 'waste' from your body. As you see the first step it was missed out by the respiratory system, second by the Digestive system as a result of your medications. Your medications were suppressing the Nature's design all the way through without realizing its intrinsic and holistic plan. As a result, you've forced

From Illness to Wellness!!!

Nature to intercept in step 3 to increase your body temperature as 'FEVER' to let the germs out.

The medications that you've taken to reduce temperature are nothing but inducing the 'SWEAT' GLANDS. This would cause a sudden change in the body, and your body.

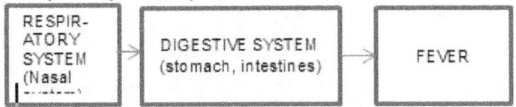

This unanticipated change in temperature will confuse the natural rhythm. It will be confused due to the fact that you're temporarily suppressing the temperature. Hence, body will be forced to reduce the temperature; however the infection is not attended by your allopathic medicines, nor have you let nature to heal you. Your body will decide to take it to the next level of giving you a much higher temperature at a later stage. Have you observed a simple phenomenon when you are sick?

You'll not feel like eating food due to lost sensations of tongue. This is a clear indication of Nature's shut-down system to stop you from eating. You'll need to **STOP RIGHT THERE. DO NOT EAT.** You're complicating the system if you eat while suffering from fever. Indeed, Nature will wait for the digestive system to perform its actions in the interim. It will look like your fever has reduced after eating food, which is not the real case. Nature has temporarily halted due to the digestive tracks, once it digests food. The fever will increase to multifold due to your ignorance.

From Illness to Wellness!!!

Indeed, Nature's design is to help you recover from ailments. **'FEVER'** is an indication of recovery process. A simple analogy…Let's assume you've identified a few armed burglars entering your house. You cannot fight alone. Hence, you'll call the police to support. The police will ask how many are there, to be equipped well ahead of the burglars to fight against them. In reality, this is what Nature is doing within your system. When it finds a lot of foreign objects in your body. It will raise the alert mechanism to throw the infections out of the body. "FEVER" is just a symptom of recovery.

You'll need to wait and listen to your body, instead of taking medications during the recovery process. It's like recovering the hardware post the crash. You'll simply execute the recovery procedure, waiting to see WINDOWS recovery done without interrupting its operations right. This is exactly what you should do. Simply observe and listen to your body. DO NOT INTERRUPT THE ALERT MECHANISM, by taking medications for FEVER. Just rest, relax and watch the whole process of Nature going on in your body. If the temperature is higher in kids or adults, there is a risk of brain getting overheated. Hence, you'll need to apply cold water pack in the forehead to avoid overheating.

Did you know small drops maketh an Ocean
Similarly, minor ailments that you had suppressed by taking temporary medications, and your ignorance had resulted in major diseases landing you

From Illness to Wellness!!!

up in hospitals as a patient permanently. Now, the Doctors won't come for rescue, they will remove all your organs, one by one!!!

Let the Nature heal you as a Dr. she knows how to take care of you. The ultimate designer knows profound ways to heal you. There is no need to interrupt in her functioning. Wouldn't you be dare to interrupt a Dr. during an operation? Just let go and heal thy self!!!
End of Session # 5.

Day 5 – Session # 6:
Marin, Don't you find the reason to identify your SKIN diseases? Let us analyze the basics of your diseases.

SKIN DISEASES

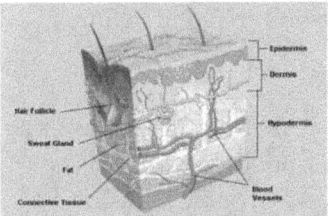Finally, it is NATURE's plan. If you recall the health chart discussed above. You've been missing out the Natural alarm system that is trying to heal you, whilst you were taking medications in STEP-1, 2 & 3 throughout to suppress it by working diametrically opposite to the natural process of healing. In simple words, you've been holding the pressure valve without releasing the pressure. Now, the final safety measure is to auto-release the safety valve without letting it explode. This is exactly happens. You didn't allow Nature to

From Illness to Wellness!!!

heal you through the process of cleasning your infection by way of SNEEZE – RUNNING NOSE – COUGH - SINUS – DIARRHEEA – FEVER.

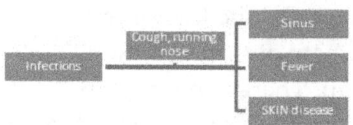

Did you see the chart indicating the multiplication of infections from sinus to fever and various skin diseases. Did you see my point, how your Doctors are treating the organs instead of the healing method as a whole. It all started as a simple running nose, wherein Nature would have healed us on its own. First, you interuppted throwing balms and other ways to avoid sneeze, running nose and cough to suppress. As a result, your infections have multiplied in to Sinus, Fever etc.

Finally the last outlet for Nature is to throw the waste in your system through the outlet of SKIN. This is exactly what you'll find as skin diseases. If you suppress it immediately using lotions, ointments without treating at the root. You end up closing the pores, which is the final outlet to let the waste out of the system. Once again think about the foolish act of holding the safety valve in a pressure cooker.

What happens if you close all the values of a pressure cooker? IT WILL EXPLODE!!! This is exactly what is happening in your body. Finally, you

From Illness to Wellness!!!

end up with chronic illness and your body loses its natural capacity to fight FOREIGN OBJECTS, as you've educated your cells and senses by the way of suppression, thus your cells are addicted to the external STIMULI to induce its natural ability to defend. This is called 'CANCER'

One of the basic diagnosis will yield all patients with SKIN diseases will have constipation.

WHAT HAPPENS TO A BOWL OF RICE KEPT CLOSED IN AN AIR TIGHT CONTAINER?
The RICE grains will spoil and you'll see it with worms coming out. If you analyze a little bit..you'll find if you have the **FIVE ELEMENTS (PANCHA BOOTHAS) such as** LAND, WATER, FIRE, AIR AND AKASH PARTICLES. THE RICE grain will be spoiled if any of these FIVE elements is not available. The irony is that NATURE is an evolutionary process, the transformation of inanimate to the animate to sublimate the negative consequences of a spoiled food. NATURE is dynamic and an evolutionary process, hence it has created life from the inanimate. Finally, the worm will feed on the rice grain as their food to survive. Eventually, after the food grain is over, these insects will eat each other, and die. Did you see my point. Nature is graceful. It is cleansing the system by removing germs either by the process of tranformation.

There is a striking resemblance in the way your germs inside the body multiplying, compared to the way you observe the above worms coming out of a dead

From Illness to Wellness!!!

body. It multiplies, and law of nature is trying to sublimate by evolution. It multiples, and eventually it will all die devoid of five elements. I believe in a similar context infections (germs) are multiplying within body by feeding in you like a parasite. If you enable your system to fight using immue system, you'll be able to heal. Instead, your allopathy medicines are treating the effect. The cause is infections due to liquidated blood which is poor in resisting. You got my point? Treat at the roots by identifying the source of it and not the branches.

This is the principle of FIVE ELEMENTS (PANCHA BOOTHA)…also indicated by Shakespeare as "DUST UNTO DUST". Your body is formed by NATURE as FIVE ELEMENTS and it will disintegrate back to the NATURE after your death. You have the measure proportion of all FIVE ELEMENTS in the body.

End of Session # 6.

From Illness to Wellness!!!

4

NATURE'S HEALING

Day 6 – Session # 7:

CHOLESTEROL ($C_{27}H_{45}OH$)

When the BAD CHOLESTEROL (LDL) increases in the BODY. It will finally form fat tumors in the BODY. Your body will generate countless nos. of good bacteria to digest your accumulated waste in the BODY. These Type A bacteria in the body will digest accumulate waste such as tumorous-fat, however it will die after digesting. The Type B bacteria formed out of Type A will be in action to clean up the Type A waste residue in the BODY. These tumors are malign or benign tumors depending on the level of infections in the respective individuals.

ALLOPATHY Medications

What happens to your pet animal after a few days of its death? There will be countless of worms formed out of its body in couple of days, ISN'T? Wouldn't it be a joke if you call the police claiming that these worms have killed your pet animal. Perhaps, no lawyer will ever argue with your case

From Illness to Wellness!!!

isn't? This is exactly what is happening in Allopathy medicines. You're ruthlessly killing all good BACTERIA, harming your whole system. Thus, as a result the damage becomes larger resulting in permanent illness as you've suppressed from the DAY I of your childhood, flaunting all the rules of the NATURE's cast. The VIRUS/BACTERIA formed in our BODY is created for all GOOD reasons, so please DO NOT mess around with it by ruthlessly killing it. These are good ones to support you in the HEALING process by the LAW OF DIVINE NATURE.

The foudation of the VEDIC HEALING is to allow these germs in the BODY to cleanse the BODY by digesting the waste. However, only care that we should take is to STOP accumulating further waste in the interim. In summary, what you've been thinking as DISEASE is not really a disease. It is an outlet to cleanup the system which is infected. If you realize this, there will be a paradigm shift in approaching your diseases differently, rather than suppressing it with short term medications. This will result in a long term consequecnces and the recoery becomes very difficult in the end. You've to befriend these diseases in the body, and realize the underlying Nature's evolutionary process.
End of Session # 7.

From Illness to Wellness!!!

Dr. Raj had learnt unique techniques from Siddhic tradition based on researching 10,000 year old literature of ancient Siddhas. This instance transformed his life…he then practiced meditation and spent years in the hills of Himalayas in silence. The Healing Tree helped him in formulating the profound and simple **"VEDIC HEALING"** methods.

> **YOU'RE ORGANICALLY CONNECTED TO MOTHER NATURE; IF YOU WILL BELIEVE..YOU'LL BE HEALED!!!**
>
> **IF YOU RESIST, YOU'LL SUFFER, WHICH BECOMES DISEASES!!!;**

"GO TEACH the WORLD"

These words echoing from deep within his heart, as he walks with a conviction to formulate workshops that would heal the conditioning of millions to help them getting out of addictions.

Dr. Guru finds his answers…in silence.

"Eureka". I'll teach the world as he starts from the hills of Coimbatore to SFO, United States. A new journey has just begun!!!

Life is just a passage of learning in the journey of consciousness towards eternity.

From Illness to Wellness!!!

Guru prepared himself for the next session...

Day 7 – Session # 8
LEARN HEALING THERAPY METHOD
DID YOU KNOW THE VACCINATION?

Almost each of you have gone through this in your life vaccination to prevent from diseases. DO you realize vaccination is a controlled dosage of POLIO virus injected to your body?

Just observe the wonderful Nature's design and its gracefulness. Once you've injected the POLIO virus into the BODY. Your child's body will prepare a solution to prevent the virus infection. It will analyze the exerternal virus as 'Good' or 'Bad'. If it determines as 'Bad', it will activate the Thymus gland with the support of organs such as liver, bone marrow, kidney will unanimously research the virus and form a solution to stop its behavior infecting your BODY. It is synonymous to you preparing a recipe for dinner.

Thus, the research scientists within your BODY will identify the virus, prepare a viable solution and finally prepare the solution & spread it in blood stream to destroy bad viruses in the main stream. These research scientists within your body are active and have the ability to destroy any bad viruses coming in. However, as you grow biologically these scientists will find it hard to get the main 'INGREDIENT' to prepare the vital medicine to

From Illness to Wellness!!!

heal within. As a result these scientists will fail to prevent the diaster. This is what is happening you become vulnerable to the diseases as you age. You've spoiled the main INGREDIENTS in blood, hence your SCIENTISTS (RB Cells) within are unable to fight it out.

There are FOUR main reasons for the loss of ingredients in BODY, resulting in reduced IMMUNITY in the BODY.

FOUR MAIN FACTORS OF DISEASES

Let's form an acronym for you to remember through your life-time.

Factors of Disease = Q2MeL.......................(1)

(You can pronounce it as Q-SQUARE-MEL)

$Q2 = Q * Q$ (Quantity & Quality of the Blood)
Me – Mind Energy
L – Quality of Life Force (Sexual Vital Fluid)

1. **Quality of blood** – Liquidated and low quality blood due to extreme addictions and extreme sensual enjoyment. Also, deficiency in the main nutrient in blood (Calcium, Zinc, Potassium etc).
2. **Quantity of blood** – 4-5 Lt is essential. There may be deficiency in blood quantity maintained. &
3. **MIND Energy** – Mind Energy is dissipated through extreme sensual pleasures, hence it will lose its power to rehabilitate your diseases. Your BODY & MIND are interlinked. Any disturbance to these layers will impact each other

From Illness to Wellness!!!

    proportinately. A healthy MIND can heal your BODY.

4. **Cell Intelligence:** Your body will lose the cell 'INTELLIGENT' system to heal thy self, & another reason is liquidated sexual vital fluid due to excessive behavior.

If you really introspect for a while after reading through the above points. Now, raise a question. Are these diseases due to an exteral agents. Perhaps because of your wrong doings so far, thus you've polluted the system and its ability to produce agents to fight the bad virus. Isn't your responsibility to realize and perform tasks in sync. with Nature? You'll be able to allow Nature healing you, if you do not mess up with the above FOUR ELEMENTS.

There is a significant harmful effect of vaccination. Once a child is vaccinated, baby's body DEFENSE mechanism will be alerted to prepare a FIGHT back system to protect itself to stop the VIRUS from infecting its territory. Hence, the child will develop IMMUNE specific to the VIRUS, however the overall IMMUNE system that a child develops as part of the normal DEVELOPMENT state through the way of breast feeding is lost. This is the BEST way to build IMMUNE system in your child by the way of brest fed milk. There is no better way to save the child. On the contrary, you apply all the vaccinations and change the biological IMMUNE system by activation its DEFENSE mechanism that are specific to VIRUS. Hence, a holistic DEFENSE mechanism that a child develops naturally is lost. The DEFENSE mechanism in your body functions as this:

From Illness to Wellness!!!

INCREDIBLE FOUR DEFENSE MECHANISM

1. **Helper** – For example. 'FLUM' is a 'helper' in your DEFENSE system that will aid in throwing out the accumulated bacteria in the BODY. Generally these are air-borne bacteria that are harmful. The first Defense mechanism uses 'FLUM' as a Helper to cleanse your respiratory system.
2. **Killer** – 'Killer' is a kind of protein prepared by your BODY DEFENSE mechanism to fight the bacteria. If Helper fails to stop the intruder, Killer will be activated by the DEFENSE system as some of the virus will intrude via FLUM into the BODY.
3. **Suppresser** – 'Suppresser' is a kind of counteractive protein that will destroy the 'Killer' protein post the above task of fight is over with the Virus. It is a kind of destructive protein to stabilize the system back to normal.
4. **Memory** – 'Memory' is your intelligence. The entire DEFENCE mechanism is restored in the brain cells.

ARTHRITIS

The four INCREDIBLE Elements of your DEFENSE mechanism functions as and when it is required. Now, after all the deliberative attempts to kill the bacteria infection in the joints, now it will start destroying tissues in the joints. This is know as **Romatade Arthritis.** If your BODY fails to produce counteractive 'Suppressor' Protein to stabilize the syste back to normal. Instead of researching about the VIRUS or BACTERIA, Our technology should change the focus in analyzing the FOUR

From Illness to Wellness!!!

INCREDIBLES mentioned above. Often you forget your lineage to the Eternal consciousness, hence all problems start escalating in your body, and mind. First, you'll need to believe in the micro-Conscousness which is the governing force in your body, and it is organically linked to the Universal conscousness (Macro Conciousness) which will supply whenever the micro conscousness demands. This is called **'FRACTION DEMANDS & TOTALITY SUPPLIES' in Vedic scriptures.** All psychological disorders are due to the excited state of MIND without realizing its lineage to the Universal consciousness.

All these diseaes are due to the disconnect between the BODY, MIND and the excessive behavior that have resulted in derailing the Orderly function which is your inherent Nature. Just like the way you change the configuration in the software application, which would no longer function the same way it does right. You'll need to do a complete analysis to even change a single line of line. Your brain has over a million nerves and there is none in the WORLD, who has completely diagnosed the human machine. It is impossible as Nature is the only designer, who could heal all condition.

Perhaps you should BELIEVE in YOURSELF and NATURE, rather than just hitting the hospitals every now and then! A simple analogy is the biological changes that a mother goes through the pregnancy is a witnessing act of mother. NATURE. What more do you want to witness…a pound of food is turned in to

From Illness to Wellness!!!

juice, blood, fat, marrow, & sexual vital fluid in your body. Is it not a wonder? Perhaps, you should BELIEVE in YOURSELF and Nature. If you analyze the FIVE Factors, you'll be able to treat any disease.

HOLISTIC HEALING

What happens to your eyes when you're angry? It will turns red isn't? Your "AKASH" energy is totally exhausted in few seconds during ANGER. As a result, your. In the above analogy of "ANGER". You've understood "HEART RATE" INCREASES, GALL BLADDER or factors increasing the chances of your anger. It is all Organically connected. A DR. is the one who can heal you holistically. There is no other way to treat you without analyzing the root causes.

Remember. **LIVER-AKASH-SALT TASTE** are all interconnected. Hence, in ancient India you would have observed pregnament women were given salty mangoes, the reason is that TASTE inhibitors will produce necessary O2 to support blood. It will give you instant energy. The SALT taste will induce AKASH shakthi in the system.

Dude, You've inherited over TEN thousand years of Wisdom as the heritage. For example..there is a saying: *"The One who eats salt will drink Water"*. This slang was used in many ocassions including the Cause and Effect system of Nature. It indicates the conversion of SALT to WATER PRANA shakti. It will induce your KIDNEY which is the source gland of WATER. Hence, you'll need to drink water to compensate WATER loss. Most of the ocassion

From Illness to Wellness!!!

"FEAR, ANXIETY" are the killer diseaes. We have already discussed the MIND power as one of the attribute for DISEASES. If you're afraid, then it will affect kidneys as you'll exhaust a lot of PRANA force, as a result water consumption is much higher. It will activate KIDNEY to supply more WATER throughout the BODY, resulting in water loss. If you observe most of the patients, their stomach will be bulged. Meaning, they have died out of fear and not because of any disease. Hence, I request each of you to be "FEARLESS" and BE BOLD.

I remember the following verssess from Mahakavi Bharathi:

**"FEAR NOT, FEAR NOT
EVEN IF THE WHOLE WORLD
IS FALLING ON THE HEAD"**

Just DROP this fear, and move on with your day to day life. Rememeber, your hospitals are infusing FEAR in the name of diseases every day. The only request is to stay tuned with the Universal consciousness & let go, surrender. Be BOLD and drive away these DISEASES.

You've mastered the first four principles of 'From Illness to Wellness':

1. Identify your 'ANATOMY';
2. Principles of Vedic Healing;
3. Transitional Therapy';

From Illness to Wellness!!!

4. Know your diseaes & **method to resolve conflict**;

CHILD Birth Deficiencies

In the next workshop, you'll learn about the CHILD birth deficiencies. Most of the deficiencies at child birth is due to the calcium deficiency in mother during the pregnancy. One fact is the deficiency of Calcium, Iron or Zinc, and the next reason is that the spoiled Calcium or Zinc in mother's blood. This is the CAUSE of a CHILD birth deficiency. I am referring to CALCIUM as an example. It may include all other deficiencies in blood. Among them are: nutrients such as glucose, fats, and amino acids; chemicals important to the body, such as sodium, potassium, and calcium; special proteins, such as fibrinogen, albumin, and various globulins that produce antibodies, which fight off viruses and other unwelcome intruders in the body; and hormones, which are regulatory substances such as insulin, and epinephrine, more familiarly known as adrenaline, which speeds up the heart rate whenever some emergency requires a greater blood flow to the muscles.

As we discussed one of the reasons such Quality & Quantity of blood, Mind factors can cause disorders in child. If a mother's mind is depressed state during pregnancy, it will impact the offspring. Hence in ancient India, every day will be a celebration to keep

From Illness to Wellness!!!

the pregnant mother happy and husband will refrain from intercourse to avoid any damage to placenta.

It is imperative to memorize the FOUR MAIN FACTORS OF DISEASES (Q2MEeL). This will help you become aware of the root causes and alievate yourself by balancing your act as appropriate.

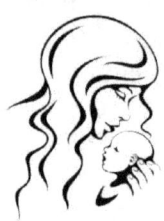

────────────Hence, I request every woman to be conscious about the FOUR MAIN FACTORS OF DISEASES to give birth to a healthy & normal CHILD to avoid any birth deficiencies & follow simple ways of living during pregnancy to give birth to a healthy child.
End of Session # 8.

From Illness to Wellness!!!

5

Vedic Healing

Day 8 – Session # 9:
Let's examine a heart related diseases. HOLE in the HEART.

Rule # 5: Follow simple ways of living

The hole in the heart can be healed through the healing method. Indeed, your blood will supply nutrient to fill the hole. Your body mechanism will await for the right nutrient, quantity available to fill the hole in the heart.

The irony is that most of the diseases are created by your own fear, and anxiety. There is no need to worry about the type of virus etc. Nature has a plan, which you should comprehend. Do not confuse or fear diseases such as CANCER. Let it be…This is exactly the reason Dr. Bruce Lipton has formulated 'Biology of Belief' to proove that Genetic disorders by no-means an indication of existing diseases in the BODY. You just have to live in the present movements with

From Illness to Wellness!!!

proper exercise, food and enjoyment in moderation through the senses. This is the successful formula for a healthy living. There is a free flow of information available in the form of TV, Internet to confuse your MIND further by infusing fear. Just ignore unwanted guests and move on with your daily life. There is no need to be paranoid with one thousand and one things happening around every day. Let Nature take care of it.

In summary, in order to remedy your heart disease, you'll need to investigate on the above FOUR main factors of diseases to heal yourself. There is no need for any medications. If the deficiency in blood is corrected, then your hole in the heart will disappear automatically.

EYE SIGHT DEFECTS

A common problem is short & long sight or Glucoma. The main reason for the Eye sight defect is due to the nutriet deficiency in the blood. The FOUR MAIN FACTORS form the cause of diseases. Wearing glasses is a stop-gap arrangement and not a permanent cure.

KIDNEY Diseases

One of the common defect is KIDNEY failure. The above FOUR factors is the reason for KIDNEY failure, as a result of deficiencies in blood. Dialysis is a stop-gap arrangement which is not a permanent cure. Even a Kidney replacement is not a viable option, as it will again spoil once it comes to your biological system.

From Illness to Wellness!!!

Indeed, you're wasting someone's kidney for no reason at all. The fact is that none of your organs can be impacted by a virus. Only the blood carrying virus impacts the Organs. Instead of treating the spare parts, you should correct the Engine Oil to repair the vehicle.

Blood Pressure

I'll explain the blood circulation process in simple terms. Your blood stream is like a train, and it stops at the Railway station. Heart is like a RAILWAY STATION & BLOOD is like a Train. The blood is purified by Liver, Kidney & bone marrow. It is formed by the conversion of food into blood. It's your heart that induces the blood pressure in the incoming blood. Let's analyze When the cell (home) picks up nutrients from the blood stream, then it will instruct via nerve center to the heart to increase the BP. If you will consider heart as a mom, and a cell as a child. Its apparent that mom will relent to the child's request. The same phenomena happnes in your heart center. Your heart will yield the cellular requests. It depends on the number of babies requesting mommy, she has to increase the work/unit, hence heart increases the BP significantly. You should remember, whenever the demand is higher with intense cellular activity, then the heart will fulfill the demand by exceeding the normal pulse rate, which is known as Blood Pressure. Often Low BP is termed as negative, which isn't true, as many monks sitting silently have had an

From Illness to Wellness!!!

extremely low BP due to lower metabolic activity, hence the demand is low for the heart to fulfill the need. For instance, if you run then the metabolism is increased, hence your BP will increase. In summary, BP is the net supply of the total demand from the cells.

Total BP (Supply) = Demand (Sum(cell1+cell2+cell3)) w/u...(1)

w/u – indicates work/unit.
The above equation indicates BP is the demand made by every cell in your biology. The demand will be proportionate to the unit work/cell. Hence, it depends on the activity that you're performing, it could be either physical or mental.

Your heart is a like a mom taking care of the needs of the cells, which are like your children. You might have observed children demanding it to their moms! This is what is called BP. Your cells are demanding to the HEART. Your family Dr. prescribes medications to suppress the children's (cells) request. As a result, the real need or requests made by the child is unknown in the medical journal, resulting in suppressing the mother, instead of understanding the reasons for the demands made by the children. Did you get my point? Eventually, your cells will die, organs will die and become dyfunctional because of the continuous medications that you've taken. Whose fault it is?

FIVE ATTRIBUTES OF WELLNESS
1. Blood Pressure

From Illness to Wellness!!!

2. Glucose
3. Oxygen &
4. Required Vitamins to heal the sickness.
5. Body consciousness

If the above FIVE attributes are in sync, then your BP will be in control and the IMMUNITY to diseases will be much higher. If any of the above attributes are spoled by your inappropriate behavior using senses, then the IMMUNITY will come down, as we discussed Four FACTORS are eseential for a healthy body, mind. Remember the formula **Q2MeL** which indicates your responsiveness to keep the sensory perceptions within limits. This is the first and the DIVINE FORMULA to remember in your life time.

$Q2 = Q * Q$ (Quantity & Quality of Blood)
Me – Mind Energy
L – Life force Quantity/Quality

The above illustration describes demand made by every cell to the HEART, thus resulting in the BP. Each cell is sending its Demand request, which is taken care by your heart. Now, think about the situation. Your DR. prescribes medications to control your BP. Alright, now what happens to the Demand of the every cell C1 to C6.

You've suppressed it by controlling the BP alone, without analyzing the demands of each CELL. As a result, you end up neglecting the DEMAND. Do you

From Illness to Wellness!!!

know what happens when you take medications for BP, does it increase over a period of time or reduces. Eventually, your Dr. will increase the dosage since your cellular demands are being rejected, you will end up increasing the dosage. A simple analogy is that..you had a car break-down. Without analyzing the source of problem you've just fixed it. It will run for another mile and then it will break down again. If you've spoiled the engine with the low grade FUEL. Your engine life will be shorter. In similar terms, you've spoiled blood and the cellular demands have increased. Without analyzing the root cause, you've temporarily suppressed the BP. This will end up in chronic illness in the end.

Did you know Dr's using BPNormal device to keep the patient's BP in a set condition during the Operation. It is true that the BP should be normal during the operation, however it is required to keep the BP normal post the surgery. The point is very simple, you should NOT control BP through medications. BP is normal, and now you've understood the reasons behind the demands made by the cell. Hence, if you suppress, your 300Million cells will be surprised to know that their heart-mom is no longer helping them. Hence, the organic unity and coordination which is Nature's intrinsic design is lost. You've fiddled around with the human machine and Nature's consciousness, as a result your cells will eventually die causing multiple organ failures.

From Illness to Wellness!!!

If you're suffering from BP. It is quiet normal, and there is no need to suppress it through the medications. Instead think about the root causes of the increased cellular demands. This is a paradigm shift in the healing, if you would like to lead a healthy life. Do not ask for the magic pills for a temporay relief, it will lead to a major disease.

LIVER DISEASES

Liver perform two main functions; It takes care of nourishing your cells by supplying nutrients from the blood, and the separated waste is moved back in to the blood stream. If you're diagnosed with diseases in liver, it indicates the problem in the nourishment of cells, meaning your cells are demanding more due to the some deficiency. You'll need to analyze the CAUSE of the demands made by the cell, rather than just suppressing the LIVER or removing the organ by surgical procedure is a sheer wastage of time, and money. This is not going to solve the problem. Your body is organically connected and by removing organ by organ will eventually leave you as a 'dead' body.

LUNG DISEASES

The air we breathe has many micro-organisms, as we discussed in the earlier chapters.

From Illness to Wellness!!!

Your nose filters in the first step and sends it to lungs. Your lungs will extract Oxygen, Hydrogen & Nitrogen from air. A simple analogy to remember, consider blood as the train and the lung as the railway station. Once the train (blood stream) arrives, passengers will board the train. Here the passengers are O2, H2 etc. Now, the train "blood stream" will distribute the O2, H2 to the houses "CELLs". It is like a power supply. Your lungs have managed to supply required O2, H2 gases exchanged to the cells for its functions. These gases will be converted to CO2 (Carbondioxide) by the CELLS in the conversion process. Now, it will go back in the reverse track from CELL to BLOOD. From Blood to nasal passage to throw out to the atmosphere.

A simple analogy as discussed before....Your liver is like a mom taking care of the necessary requirements from the children "BABY". When the demand is more, which indicates your children are doing something excessive or perhaps a requirement. It depends on the situation. Now, if you're treating LUNGS alone for the diseases such as 'ASTHMA, SINUS, COUGH, TB' etc. which indicates you're suppressing the mother without being able to help the children (cells). These children (cells) will suffer, eventually leading to lack of coordination from the mother, as a result it will die out of conflict, resulting in major Organ failure. Hence, the first point of your analysis should be the cells to understand its behavior and the increase in

From Illness to Wellness!!!

"DEMAND". Further these factors that are attributing to the "DEMAND". Instead, if you suppress "LUNGS" by taking medications, it will result in thousands of cells being impacted. For example. If your Kidney is infected, then LUNGS will step up to supply more air to Kidneys to heal by itself as per the Natural proces. Did you see you are interrupting the natural healing process by your short-term medications.

Your LUNGS are like a "AIR FILTER and supplier" which takes care of needs of millions of cells to function by supplying O2, H2 etc. The damage to the organ is not by the itself, indeed the CAUSE is somewhere. This is where you'll need to diagnose, not in the specific ORGAN. By stripping every ORGAN from the body is going to leave you a DEAD body eventually. A deteriorating LUNGS will indicate the increased demand to supply air (O2, H2) to the cells. Hence, you should analyze the CAUSE of the increase in the requirements from the cell. Perhaps you should learn from treating it at the root instead of the branches.
End of Session # 9.

From Illness to Wellness!!!

6

INFECTIONS

Day 9 – Session # 10:
YOUR BODY is going through a constant change. The white blood cells are rejuvenated every 13 days & the red blood cells are rejuvenated every 120 days. Your body is made up of cells. Appx. 300 Million cells are rejuvenated in the system / minute.

INFECTIONS IN KIDNEY

The same analogy as discussed before. Your blood stream is "TRAIN" and the KIDNEY is the "RAILWAY STATION". Your KIDNEY will separate nutrients from WATER and transfer it to the TRAIN which is the Blood stream to support various cell functioning. Your cells will utilize the nutrients in WATER, and then send the extracts in the reverse track back to the blood stream. Every single will send the extract 'quanta of urine' back to the blood stream, which is collected in the urinary bladder.

You have to assume "KIDNEY" as a mother who supplies WATER to every CELL, which is her CHILD. When the demand from the children increases, mom

From Illness to Wellness!!!

will have to work harder than before. As a result KIDNEY is affected .

What is point in replacing **KIDNEY?** It is going to get a similar DEMAND sooner or later! The newer KIDNEY will also be impacted soon. Hence, the root cause is to analyze the CELLULAR requests for increased DEMAND in WATER requirements in CELL structure. You cannot cure by simply stripping out KIDNEY from your biology. Your Kidney will supply water to the heart, hence if there is an impact to the Kidneys, your heart will also be impacted, and in similar terms your lungs will supply air to the heart. If your lungs are impacted, your heart will be impacted too.

In summary, what you should understand is that there is nothing wrong in the Organs and there is no need to cure the organs. Indeed the cure is required to the cells that have increased the DEMAND. A real cure/healing will be analyzing the root causes of the increased DEMAND and treating it at the roots. Please remember treating individually a the Organ level is not appropriate and not a cure at all.

End of Session # 10.

From Illness to Wellness!!!

Day 10 – Session # 11:

DIABETES

Glucose - Just remember the story that we talked about…your cell as a "HOME" with the bloodstream as a "ROAD." Food is digested in the small intestines, and it is assimilated into blood through liver. Your food content comprises of carbohydrates, proteins, vitamins & fiber. The carbohydrate is converted to glucose (sugar). Now, the CELL's will open up to accept the nutrients such as Calcium, Magnesium, Ion, & sodium from Blood. However, CELL do not accept glucose directly. Hence, it will analyze it as good sugar or bad sugar first as part of the process.

A good sugar is the one which is due to a proper digestion of food. If food is not digested properly in the intestines, it turns into bad sugar. In this process of segregation, cells will raise questions to the sugar whether its bad or good. It will further send it to the pancreas to investigate good vs. bad. If pancreas determines it to be good, it will substitute with "INSULIN". If it is a bad sugar, then there will not be any substitute.

From Illness to Wellness!!!

STEP 1 – Extract SUGAR (glucose) from food through the carbohydrate

STEP 2 – Determine GOOD or BAD using pancreas prior to assimilation into Cell.

STEP 3 – Pancreas will determin GOOD vs. BAD. Good will be Quality Checked, and substitute with INSULIN, which is further passed on for cell function. BAD WILL BE sent to URINARY bladder.

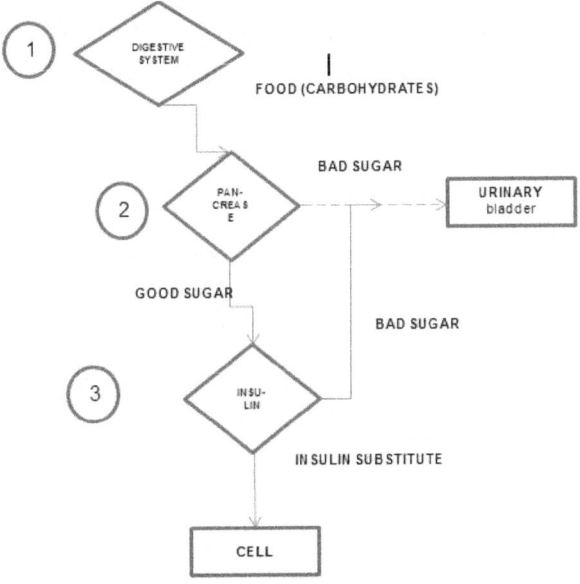

Here pancreas is the Quality Controller who determines the good. Vs. bad sugar.

$C_6 H_{12} O_6$ - The above formula indicates Glucose. It is known as Isomer. It refers to the multiple sub-constituents.

From Illness to Wellness!!!

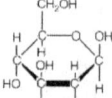 The above illustration is the atomic structure of glucose. Perhaps the DIABETIC analysis done will indicate the overall level of sugar, but cannot give you a clear indication of the different types of glucose level. Only IR STUDY, UV SPECTRUM study will get you a detailed analysis of types of glucose to determine blood glucose level. PLASMA GLUCOSE LEVEL is different from the sugar level in blood. Therefore, DIABETES does not indicate anything wrong with the PANCREAS in secreting INSULATION.

DID You get my point? The lack of insulin is due to the quantity of bad sugar in your body. And the bad sugar is due to the result of the indigested food. Now, you tell me is it prudent to identify the source or treating the cause? The source is food & your habit of eating food holistically!!!!

When you were a child, you were able to digest food completely. Hence. The sugar is mostly good sugar in children. When the cells extract sugar via pancreas from blood, excess will be sent back to the blood stream. For example. If your cells are expecting 200 units of sugar. If the intake is 500 units, then the cells will reject 300u. the net sum of the left over sugar 300u will the consolidated into Glycogen, say about 1000u sugar, which will be stored in the muscle fibres, BRAIN & LIVER. It will be used when needed.

From Illness to Wellness!!!

The first level of bad sugar is formed in children when mom's force them to eat without children are really hungry. As a result, the bad sugar level increases.

What happens to the bad sugar which are sent back to the blood without a substitute "INSULIN". It cannot be assimilated to CELLs as discussed. Now, it will be accumulated in the blood as bad sugar. Finally, your body determines to eliminate the bad sugar through urine. So, remember whenever you are subjected to the URINE tests and if the DR. says you have excessive SUGAR levels. Do indicate to him, Doc: *"These are all bad sugars and our body is intelligent enough to send it out. There is no need to be paranoid by it."*

Let's say you'll need **300u** of sugar for the metabolic routine. What happens if there is a deficit due to an increased bad sugar. In total 500u of sugar, let's say 200u is good and 300u is bad. You'll have a deficit of sugar levels by 100u isn't? remember we talked about 'Glygogens' which are good-sugar packets that will supply on-need basis. Now. Your body will instruct pituitary gland will secrete fluids known as 'ACTH', which will activate adrenalin gland. This will further instruct usage of the Glycogens stored in the brain, liver and muscles. Hence. You'll not feel the deficit. However, if this continues by assuming you aren't taking good food, resulting in excessive bad-sugar. Then, at some point even the Glycogen's cannot fulfill your need. You will be deficient of required sugar levels. It's like losing fuel in the car, even the

From Illness to Wellness!!!

reserve levels are gone as the Pituitary gland will instruct cells about the lack of glucose supply. As a result you'll feel giddiness. This is the indication of the 'reserve' levels have been completely utilized. As a result, your cells will not get enough intake of glucose. Hence, your cells will feel tired soon without required intake of glucose levels, and the reserves have dried too. You'll feel tired often if you're DIABETIC.

URINE TESTS TO DETERMINE HIGH/LOW SUGAR LEVELS. In reality the quanta of Glycogens used by your body. If there is no "RESERVE" then it is called LOW sugar. Perhaps, medical terms are a little confusing as they determine HIGH/LOW based on the Urine tests. It depends if the test is conducted in the Urine after the passing out bad-sugar, then it will indicate the Low sugar level. On the contrary, if the Urine test is done even before a patient has urinated, then it will indicate an increased sugar level, They will immediately term it as HIGH sugar level. This is not the exact representation of your sugar levels in the blood.

Infact, the blood sugar levels will vary depending on the requirements from the cell. It cannot be determined someone with high/low sugar levels in one tests as it depends on the situation and the cell's demand.

A simple analogy:

From Illness to Wellness!!!

You've invited your colleagues for dinner. Say around. FIVE and you were surprised to see the TEN including your colleagues friends arrived for dinner. You'll need to prepare food for TEN, which was initially planned for FIVE. It may vary. Sometimes your family members may eat out, resulting in preparing food for just TWO. Would you complain that you mom is not preparing enough food? As the quantity of intake varies every day, so does the sugar levels in the body.

The increase in SUGAR levels depends on the environment also. For example. If you find a snake passing body. Your alert system will produce sugar to keep it ready to fight poison, hence the sugar levels will increase temporarily to support your cells to throw the poison out. It will be back to the normal once you feel you're out of danger. It's very dynamic, and cannot be mesaured. You cannot DETERMINE HIGH/LOW based on conducting tests on a given DAY. It is good to use INSULIN in emergency, not on a regular basis.

End of Session # 11.

From Illness to Wellness!!!

Day 11 – Session # 12

Rule # 5 – Discover simple ways of living
What happens to the INSULIN shots that you've taken?

Let's analyze the above process. Let's say a patient is unconscious due to HIGH sugar levels…say about 400u. Your pancreas will inform that it is all BAD SUGAR, hence it didn't substitue with required INSULIN for cell function, despite having required INSULIN. It will not substitute for BAD SUGAR. Now, your insulin shots will enforce PANCREAS to substitute 'INSULIN' for all 400units of BAD SUGAR, defying its own intelligence. It is like a duplicate certificate for bad SUGAR to fool the internal system which is functioning in absolute precision. You've changed the system. It's like you've changed a software program in a critical application without identifying the root cause. It will be a temporary fix, resulting in a major bug in the application. These INSULIN shots are inhibitors that will enforce your PANCREAS to certify BAD SUGAR as 'GOOD' to fool the cellular intelligence. A simple question that I'd ask is that whether the dosage in DIABETIC's is increasing or reducing. It's an organized crime and politics to make someone feel like a patient.
As a result, the BAD SUGAR which has been forced to assimilate into the cell biology will eventually affect

From Illness to Wellness!!!

cells, organs etc. and the entire system will be dyfunctional as a result of increased BAD SUGAR LEVELS. Eventually your PANCREAS will become dyfunctional, and all other ORGANS will follow suit. This is happening due to the medications on a daily basis that you're taking for maintain SUGAR levels. Slowly you'll have eye defects due to increased dosage, then followed by KIDNEY. However, all Doctors will uninanimously point at you saying
...*'You haven't kept the SUGAR levels in control'*

The bottom line is that you should not control SUGAR levels. It is a varying attribute depending on the cell function as discussed. If you control, it will result in myriads of diseases, leading to multiple diseases.

End of Session # 12.
*

From Illness to Wellness!!!

Day 12 – Session # 13: Know the consequences of taking unncessary medications

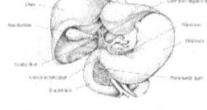

Gall Bladder

The BILE fluid is stored by the GALL BLADDER, which is essential for digestion & it will separate 80% Cholestrol from food. Just imagine the consequences of blindly removing the '**GALL BLADDER**'. Then, who will store required '**BILE**' fluid. How do you anticipate DIGESTION post removal of GALL BLADDER. What non-sense is this? Nature has a perfect and organic way of dealing with the physiology. And the Human minds seem to have complicated it totally.

Tumor in Uterus

One of the primary functions of UTERUS in women is a GOD's gift to humanity for conception and the baby grows here. Its secondary function is to removing waste from the body.

Hence, imagine the blind consequences of removing Uterus. As a result of removal, your sweat glands, urinary bladder will be overloaded to excrete excess waste that were part of Uterus's responsibliites. Hence, its unit work increases. It has become a fashion statement to remove Uterus as we hear every woman discussing it in pride. Please be aware, Uterus removal is not necessary. DO NOT PANIC what your Doctors say. They are the organized

From Illness to Wellness!!!

politicians. I believe a law should me amended to **STOP** removal of **'ORGANS'**. It is like killing someone in your home! You don't have any right to kill someone in your home as per law, the same applies here as well. Doctors have decorated their profiles with inflated bank balances with pride in annoncing the number of successful surgical procedures. Only GOD knows how many successful and healthy patients are alive post surgical methods. It's the same old joke:

"OPERATION SUCCESSFUL BUT PATIENT IS DEAD" If they want to practice surgical procedures, perhaps they can try out in their own family before proceeding to others.

Appendicites

It's easy. If you have appendix problems, your Doctor will advise for a quick surgery to remove. This is all they've studied their whole life to remove every Organ in your body. This is not our ancient wisdom or traditional healing methods of Indian system. Perhaps, this is all western medicine from the school of Aristotle. We have submerged our ancient wisdom, the wisdom of Bodhi Dharma, siddhas that were very profound healing methods. We should go back to our history in identifying profound healing methods. Let's analyze the functions of Appendix. It helps in removing waste from the body. It helps in maintain **'Equilibrium'** in the body. If your Appendix is removed, the body

From Illness to Wellness!!!

balance will be lost forever. It will be apparent if you watch a patient post removal of appendix, he/she will not be walk uphill with required balance. If someone tells me that there is a Organ that is of no use, which indicates that the creator has done it by mistake. Can it be true? GOD has created the ultimate physiology in pattern, precsion & regularity in everything from the smallest atom to the galaxies. You're organically connected. It cannot be possible that GOD has created something within you without a purpose. It is because of a few foolish medical experts that you end up loosing an Organ. Perhaps, we should find an alternative medicate without having to relent to the surgical procedures of removing an Organ.

Did you know the reason why SUGAR patients legs are amputated?
Remember the earlier discussions, we discussed about the GOOD vs. BAD SUGAR. The INSULIN medicines prescribed will certify the BAD SUGAR as GOOD and enforce PANCREAS to certify the 'BAD SUGAR' to assimilate it for cell functions. Hence, your blood stream carrying BAD SUGAR will destroy all ORGANS one-by-one. There is a difference in insulin tablets vs. insulin shots. The insulin intake through tables will not directly mix into the blood, as per the process it will go through the PANCREAS to be certified, prior to mixing with the blood for supplying it to cells. However, insulin shots directly certify BAD sugar as GOOD directly in te blood stream. Whichever cell/organs receiving this sugar blocks will be completely destroyed. It's a pity that you're flaunting with the LAWS of Nature to

From Illness to Wellness!!!

destory your own body in the end. Nature is merciful till the end, death is the ultimate relief from all your sufferings. It is intended for protecting you if you suppress all its natural healing methods through the way of your discovery. Whoever using the thes INSULIN SHOTS will definetly face a multiple ORGAN failure over a period of time. One more information is that these INSULIN sold is extracted from animals.

Eventually due to regular intake of INSULIN SHOTS, you're foot will start numbing as the cells will decay. As a result, your Doctor. Will further advice you to amputate it as early as possible. This is their technology, and blessing for following their prescribed medications. You've to move very far away from these Doctors. Perhaps, just stay atleast a few hundred miles away from the hospitals. They are good for accidents and medical emergencies, not for the regular medications that will damage your Organs. In the end you'll be amputating Organs, one after the other!

Did you get my point? What are you wondering about...Listen, there is no disease called DIABETES. It is your Doctors wild imagination. The only remedy that you should follow is to eat healthy food to digest carbohydrate completely through the intestines, thus helping Nature do the remaining process of conversion. Your resonsibility is to eat when you're only hungry, then follow a good meal practices without dumping garbage food. Take a light vegetarian meal that is soulful and tasteful. It will

From Illness to Wellness!!!

rejuvenate your BODY, MIND AND SPIRIT. If you want to lead a healthy life, just eat a good Vegetarian meal to heal your body, mind and spirit. **Nature loves Veggies.** The basic rule is to digest carbohydrates completely, leaving no room for BAD sugar. All GOOD sugar will help you build enough day-to-day requirements of cells and in addition it will build the reserve "GLYCOGENS" to use it in times of need.

The irony is that DIABETES is not due to the eating sweets or candies. Indeed, it is due to the BAD SUGAR and your responsibility in eating a complete light quality meal that is digestable. It will translate into GOOD SUGAR. Hence, there is no need to quit eating your favoirte chocholates, candies, or pastries. In our healing method, you should eat it to build GOOD SUGAR, in order to increase the GOOD SUGAR levels to the required levels. Hence, you do not need to remain starving, instead, just eat healthy food depending on your appetite. Eat health in moderation is the secret formula for defeating this disease. I believe these so called Doctors are trusting Aristotle, much beyond their own bodies and have the best memories in the WORLD with no realization of self or others.

***

From Illness to Wellness!!!

Rule # 6 Healing Method

In summary, all you've to understand is that you'll need to identify the root causes of your illness, treating it at the root. You'll need to identify the reasons for the CELLS demanding higher glucose, or higher H20 or 02 resulting in increased supply & work for the respective ORGANS. HEART, LUNGS, LIVER, KIDNEY & PANCREAS. Hence, instead of treating it at the ORGAN, you should consider a holistic approach.

You should also understand SUGAR level variation is not an immediate disease and/or BP is not you should treat by taking medications. If you take medications over a period of time, it will result in multiple negative consequences of impacted ORGANS as a result. Finally, as an ultimatum your Doctor will remove the ORGAN by organ leaving you a DEAD body.

As you've understood. A perfect healthy male will have required 'GLYCOGENS'. This is the reserve glucose stored in the muscle fibre, brain as discussed. When someone meets with an accident and unconscousness, it will help in rescue by providing required glucose to support survival. A perfectly healthy male/female will have required reserves, which are GLYCOGENS & used during the emergency.

Hence, my recommendations to you is to request you for eating well and healthy in moderation depending on the appettite. Do not over eat, eat in moderation

From Illness to Wellness!!!

and respect your inner system with 300Million cells coordination in the process of digestion and transformation of nutrient from blood to organs and excretory process. Is it not a wonder?
Next time, when you're having dinner. I'll join, let's eat consciousnessly, thus aware of the intrinsic qualities of mother. Nature playing through you. You are no way lesser than the Universe. The entire mechanism of the Universe, forces, quantum mechanics...particle theory. It is all there in your biology as micro biology. Just feel thankful to GOD. Hold and feel the food, thank the Eternal Conscousness for her love and gratitude.

YOUR DIABETES could be either due to the deterirated PANCREAS or perhaps DIGESTIVE problems. If it digestive reasons, then you should streamline the food practices as discussed. You'll be able to reduce all medications in step-by-step method. **Enjoy the meal!!!** There is no disease to follow except for the Doctors & Scientists those who are inventing it. There is no correlation between 'SUGAR FREE' tablets. It's just another marketing gimmics to fool you.

Thyroid

'THROID' is due to calcium deficiency in blood. There is a certain quantity of calcium required in the blood. The Calcium in blood is segregated to 1. GOOD & 2. BAD which indicates a completely digested calcium as good. BAD Calcium is inadequately digested calcium.

From Illness to Wellness!!!

Increased level of calcium in blood: If the calcium quantity is high in blood, then your Thyroid gland will function to segregate excess "bad" calcium to the bones. Hence, your bones will be impacted. This may decay your bones. Your Doctor's will indicate that the Thyroid gland as a culprit causing impact to the bone, with no claims to their accusations as ever. Perhaps they'll accuse Nature at some point for everything without realizing the Nature within. Hence, you should realize the quality of calcium in blood is the reason for damage, and not the thyroid gland.

Reduced level of calcium in blood: A reverse phenomenon happnes if the calcium level decreases. Then, your para-thyroid gland will extract calcium from the bones. The bottom line is these are defeciencies in quality of calcium blood, not a deficiency in the gland itself.

Your muscles contraction is controlled by the thyroid glands. Your muscle fibre will require calcium for contraction, which is being supplied by thyroid glands. If quantity of calcium is below par in the blood, your thyroid gland will not be able to function effectively to support the muscle functions. It will result in contraction but cannot retract back to normal, hence your skin will shrink, but not retract back to the normal. You'll turn slim with significant loss of weight which is not healthy with contracted muscles.

From Illness to Wellness!!!

Your thyroid gland will need sodium for muscle contraction. As a result, your muscles will contract but will not retract back. Hence, the calcium deficiences in blood will resulti n impacting thyroid gland. As a result, you'll either gain or lose weight considerably. It's like the functions performed by thyroid gland such as contractions / expansion of muscles will depend on the quantity of calcium. Calcium deficiencies in blood will lead to poor quality of work, which is contraction/expansion of muscles, resulting in over weight or considerable weight loss.

The bottom line is that you'll need to understand THYROID is due to the calcium, sodium deficiencies in blood and not the gland itself. Hence, by improving the quantity of food and your ability to digest food completely would result in producing more "good" Calcium without any medications.

There is an incorrect notion that Milk is the only source of Calcium. Just think, if Cow is eating fresh leaves, it is able to convert it to milk. The same logic should apply for us as well. If you eat green leafy vegetables, spinach, your body will separate required calcium from food. You should take a lot of vegetables, spinach and milk to increase calcium intake.

End of Session # 13.

**

From Illness to Wellness!!!

Day 12 – Session # 14. Belive yourself & Nature who is the only Master Healer.
Last but not least, I am going to teach you about the convictions of truth based on the Hindu mythology. A few videos to watch. Sit back & relax. We have discussed about Diseases and the incorrect medications that is further agravating the condition. The fact is that you should hold on to the convictions of truth. As you realize Nature is the '**Cause and Effects**' system, It is apparent God is descending as results.

As Bhagvad Gita says:
'I'll reveal myself to you as results'

The above statement indicates the cause and effects theory as Nature itself manifesting as results. If you do it incorrectly, confronting the laws of Nature, you'll end up in pains. **What happens if you do over eat?** You will have to face the consequences of an upset stomach. This is a simple example and no need for any philosophy. You will need to realize the senses by paying attention to the situation. The emerging thoughts, actions, work, sex, and rest etc.

You should counsel yourself; analyze the limited happiness created by these senses, with the limitations of senses. If you need eternal bliss, the only way is to transcend the senses. Enjoyment in moderation.

From Illness to Wellness!!!

Rule # 7 Prevention is better than Cure

What is the point in worrying about the results? By the time you're worrying, the past instance is gone. Either way you have to be prepared for a result and it will come as per the Nature's Divine justice. It is the time right now, to analyze your painful sensations, and contemplate and counsel by holding on to center **'The Truth'** itself. This will heal your condition & eleavte to the higher plane of life.

Often Zen techniques portray moment to moment awareness in every action, which is indicated in Bhagvat Gita as the 'Karma Yoga' by practicing action in the state of detached attachment in total awareness. Tell them about the 7 rules with profound healing techniques and help them achieve what they want

Guru thanks Dr.Raj for teaching the simple and profound techniques to help in succeed...The FOUR MAIN FACTORS that you've analyzed is very profound. The formula Q2MeL (which is pronounced as Q-SQUARE-MEL) is helpful to remind yourself on the primary factors. Now, if you observe a patient who has met with an accident, the very first thing Doctors will do is to compensate his blood loss. And second with the nutrients such as Glucose water or Sodium Chloride to support cell functions.

Did you observe? The hospitals have saved a number of lives through blood transfusion & Glucose alone. Did they treat anyone Organ by Organ?

From Illness to Wellness!!!

These are the four primary factors that you will need to watch out for. Did you observe a simple phenomenon? If you go to a Doctor. With a pain in the eyes or joints, he/she will inject medicine to relieve the pain. The fact is that blood will carry the medicines to the respective cells in the Organ that will take to cure it isn't? In reality a specific nutrient that a group of cells expecting in an organ is not available in blood. This is the root cause of diseases.

In a similar term, hairfall…is also mainly due to the a specific nutrient deficiency in blood. The hair cells are perhaps expecting these deficient nutrient in blood, but not getting its proper dosage or perhaps the intelligent mechanism in cells to rejuvenate hair follicles is lost. For all reasons that you may summarize, try & analyze the "**Q2MeL**" formula to identify the root causes. You'll be able to comprehend truth that the diseases are not there in the Organ, it is there in the blood due to deficiencies. All diseases such as tumor, kidney stones, sinus, asthma, cough, gasterontology, arhritis, gastric trouble, sexual disorders, thyroid, diabetes, AIDS, Cancer, eye defects etc.

Mostly sexual disorders are due to excessive sexual behavior at a young age. Perhaps you should avoid excessive behavior. Now you should balance it via proper food & regular practices to increase life force, you'll regain the lost energy. In addition to the Q2MeL as primary factors, there are secondary factors that you'll need to understand.
    1.   Impact to the intelligence mechanism (cell),

From Illness to Wellness!!!

2. Imprints in the Subconscious mind as conditioning,
3. Pancha boothas (Five Elemets) proportion,
4. Child birth deficiencies &
5. Genetic Disorders/Imprints.

There could be many other factors for diseases, however we would restrict to the formalae **"Q2MeL"** as the primary factor with the secondary factors discussed above. If you want further summarize in ONE STATEMENT. You'll be surprised to hear the main reason for all diseases is:
"LOW - QUALITY OF BLOOD"

Always remember Allopathy medicines will give you temporary relief. Al right, but DO NOT CONTINUE. It is good for an emergency but not on a daily basis. Now, you should try the following practices to purify BLOOD. Yoga, Breathing practices, Medication, Accu Pressure, Neuro Therapy, Mudras, Reiki, Pranic Healing, Touch Healing, Magneto Therapy which are safe as they are natural methods **to PURIFY BLOOD. The ACU PRESSURE** techniques are very profound, as they remove the blockages and enhance the flow of blood, air, heat circulation & BIO-MAGNETIC circulation in the body to **HEAL THY SELF!!!** You should understand defeciencies in the blood. Ok.

HOW DO YOU PURIFY YOUR BLOOD?
Let us see the possible healing…& Nature medicines:
1. LAND - FOOD will be converted to BLOOD
2. AIR – Nitrogen, Oxygen

From Illness to Wellness!!!

3. WATER – Hydrogen
4. HEAT - Physical excercises will provide heat to the body & blood &
5. AKASH – Your blood has akash particles which will be nourished during sleep to rejuvenate.

Vedic Secret Propounded

You'll need to learn the following secrets of Vedas as explained in our ancient scriptures:
1. Vedic Secret **LAND** # 1 – Digesting food that you eat positively
2. Vedic Secret **WATER** # 2 – Digesting water
3. Vedic Secret **FIRE** # 3 – Breathing ways to inhale air for nutrients such as sodium, magnesium etc.
4. Vedic Secret **AIR** # 4 – Physical exercices to provide enough work/heat to the body
5. Vedic Secret **AKASH** # 5 - SLEEP.

If you are taking required quantity of food without over heating, then your body will absorb radiations from ISOTOPES, thus enhancing its blood with all requried nutrients. A healthy blood will result in a healthy BODY. Once your bone marrow identifies reuqired nutrients in blood, it will starts its process of new blood cells in 120 Days. This will keep all your ORGANS healthy. Your bone marrow will prepare an essense that will heal your body entirely. There is no additional medicine required for anything from any other sources. Your body is a temple where it has the automous system to heal you holistically. There are FIVE POINTS THAT YOU WILL NEED TO FOLLOW:
    1. FOOD,

From Illness to Wellness!!!

2. WATER,
3. AIR,
4. WORK &
5. REST

Follow a simple routine:

FIVE POINT STRATEGY

FOOD, REST, INTERCOURSE, WORK & THOUGHTS. If You follow a simplified routine with limits in above five elements will heal you totally. Have you observed a simple phenomenon? You get instant energy from food, how is it possible> as the food assimilation in your body takes atleast two hours. The truth is that taste buds will absorb respective taste of sour, bitter, salty, sweet, sour. The taste buds will convert it to oxygen through liver (manneral) to distribute to the cells.

Transformation of Taste

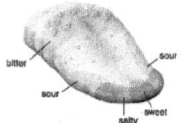

1. SALT – When you taste 'SALT' in food, it will transform in to "PRANA SHAKTHI" & distribute throughout the BODY.
2. SOUR– An excessive utlization of liver will need transformation of sour taste to AKASH
3. SPICE, BITTER & SWEET.

What happens to the food you eat?
4. STEP 1 – Food that you eat becomes is crushed and becomes 'JUICE'.

From Illness to Wellness!!!

5. STEP 2 – It reaches the intestines. It becomes 'BLOOD'. Extract SUGAR (glucose) from food through the carbohydrate, determine GOOD vs. BAD based on PANCREAS which will approve & substitute with 'INSULIN' & it will finally assimilate with BLOOD Determine GOOD or BAD using pancreas prior to assimilation into Cell.
6. STEP 3 – FAT is extracted from food
7. STEP 4 – FLESH is extracted from food
8. STEP 5 - BONES
9. STEP 6 – Calcium is extracted & assimilated to the BONE MARROW &
10. STEP 7 – Finally it becomes SEXUAL VITAL FLUID which is the source of LIFE FORCE. Millions of LIFE FORCE particles are formed from the VITAL FLUID. Hence, it is your responsibility to maintain a certain minimum quantity & quality of the sexual vital fluid.

From Illness to Wellness!!!

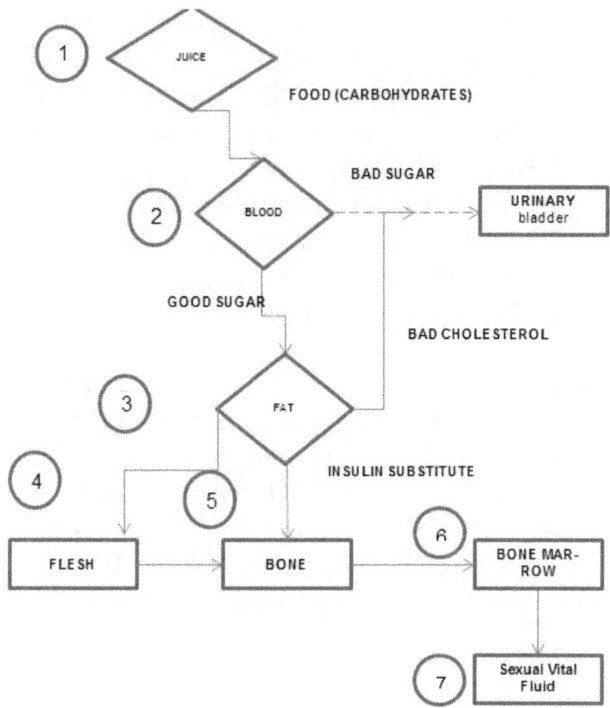

"FOOD IS MEDICINE" as ancient scriptures describe. This is true when it is taken in moderation. An excess will leave undigested food in intestines, causing more BAD SUGAR, CHOLESTEROL. Hence, eating FOOD is a social act and you should act with absolute responsibility and awareness. Just remember, your 300 Million cells are in action when you eat to assimilate into blood, cells for its functioning.

From Illness to Wellness!!!

If you're a '**NON-VEGETARIAN**' eating RED meat, please avoid it in steps over a period of time. It has multiple negative consequences as it required longer to digest food, and secondly the food that you eat becomes your body. It will result in tranforming into MIND too…You'll become vulnerable mentally and physically. Hence, avoid it in steps. A good vegetarian meal comprising of pulses, grain & vegetables is sufficient for your metabolism. Dr. Ornish has extensively talked about the harmful effects of NON-VEGETARAN food. There are poisonous harmones secreted by these animals before the slaughter, Hence, these harmones will be extremely poisonous to you as well. "STOP EATING NON-VEG FOOD". Above all, it will increase the imprints assimilated through the animals, hence it will not be viable for you. While you're trying to sublimate your current karma's, adding burden to your cells is not a wise idea, isn't? Think about it!

When you eat, be totally aware and conscious of the food that you want to digest completely. Eat slowly, chew completely and then assimilate food. DO NOT GULP it or DRINK WATER or EAT in a HURRY. Do NOT overeat. All of that would attribute to the BAD CHOLESTEROL, SUGAR etc. Eat when you're angry and not by TIME. Eat as per your BIOLOGICAL clock, when the cells need it, eat slowly and conscoiusnessly. Give some respect to **300 Million** children (cells) within you. You've to socialize with your cells to enable complete DIGESTION and assimilation of food into your physiology.

From Illness to Wellness!!!

The first ELEMENT is LAND. FOOD is related to the 'LAND', which is one of the FIVE ELEMENTS. The food that you eat contains minerals, carbohydrates, sugar, protein, vitamin, minerals. These are related to 'LAND' which is one of the PANCHA BOOTHA. The second element is WATER. The kidney will segregate required oxides from water, which is related to the third element 'WATER'.

The Third element is FIRE. The heat energy is generated in the BODY, when your body is engaged in work. Hence, work is absolutely essential in moderation. Next, AIR you breathe also supplies energy, hence AIR is also a medicine as you extract Nitrogen, Oxygen from AIR, which passes via Lungs and mixes in blood. This is related to the second element of pancha bootha.

The final and the fifth element is AKASH or energy particles which is absorbed when your are in deep sleep. You'll need to eat required quantity of food in order to ensure all FIVE elements are absorbed by your physiology. If you over eat, air, fire energy will become inadequate causing deficiencies in blood. The root cause of all diseases is due to the improper DIGESTION. If food is not digested, it will lead to bad sugar, cholestrol etc. If you learn the ways to absorb five elements as indicated above, then your blood will be very pure with all required nutrients.

One of the task of bone marrow is to rejuvenate blood every 48 hours, as soon as the required nutrients are available. All your RBC is completely

From Illness to Wellness!!!

rejuvenated in 120 days. If you are able to provide required nutrient to 'BONE MARROW', it will rejuvenate high quality 'BLOOD'.

In summary, if you are able to get required quantity of nutrients from the above FIVE ELEMENTS, then your BLOOD will be extremely PURE. The first approach in our HEALING method is to ensure the 'BONE MARROW' gets its nutritient requiremetns to rejuvenate 'BLOOD'. TASTE buds can quickly turn food into Oxygen required for metabolism. The food that you eat should have required SPICES. SALT, SPICE, SUGAR etc.

YOU CAN CURE BP by SALT INTAKE

The irony is that if you have BP, your Dr's will advice avoiding SALT totally. Al right, even after ten years, if you have avoided SALT, does it solve the problem? You're still continuing with the BP isn't? has it solved your problems? The fact is that SALT increases BP true, but Nature's design could have a reason to it. Let's analyze.

Ok. Let us see what happens when you TASTE SALT. The moment you taste a pinch of salt through your taste buds will convert it to 'WATER' current & activate the KIDNEY. Kidney will purify blood by extracting the waste from blood, to excrete waste through URINE. During this process, your BLOOD will be liquidated. Hence, HEART will pump blood with a higher pressure than usual.

Now see NATURE's design and DR.s point of VIEW.

From Illness to Wellness!!!

NATURE DESIGN is to instruct your kidney to purify blood when you take SALT. And your DR's view is to suppress the reaction of heart in the process of blood purification & hence they term eating salt is BAD. It has a purpose if you understand and view it holistically. Now, you'll be able to comprehend SALT is good if taken in moderation to purify blood. If it is totally avoided, you'll be devoid of SALT, thus halting the blood purification process. You've messed up the natural rhythm causing significant problems. Hence, I request you to take required intake of SALT to avoid further conequences to the ORGANS such as KIDNEY and HEART.

You should remember the relation between the emotions and Organs. If you're afraid – 'fear, anxiety' will impact kidneys. If you are angry, you'll impact DIGESTIVE system as you're exhausting PRANA shakthi. Hence, if you eat with anger you'll not digest. Please realize the emotions and its relation to each of the organs. If you are subjected to emotional moods, DO NOT EAT! It will lead to BAD cholesterol, Sugar etc.

YOU CAN CURE DIABETES by SUGAR INTAKE

The moment you taste SUGAR, Your 'LAND' current throughout the body and it will activate spleen. You'll need glucose for metabolic

From Illness to Wellness!!!

routine. If your cells are starved for glucose, it will become tired soon and eventually lead to deteoriating health.

The SUGAR that you taste via taste BUDS is different from the Glucose that is assimilated into blood stream. The SUGAR TASTE will activate intestines. Once you activate INTESTINES, SUGAR will be extracted from the blood. If you suppress it without taking enough SUGAR intake, will result in reduced SUGAR assimilation into cells, resulting in frequent tired frequently. Also, the SUGAR assimilation is not taking place, thus resulting in wasted SUGAR from the BODY. You know the loss of SUGAR will lead to feeling extremely tired. If you've adequate SUGAR in BLOOD, it will feed all CELL & thus ORGANS will be healthy.

There is another myth, Dr's have attributed RICE as the reason for excessive SUGAR intake. Ok, then why would North Indians suffer from Diabetes, despite taking Chapathi in their daily meal? The irony is that, Dr's in North INDIA are advocating eating RICE to their patients. Ultimately, each of you have been termed as 'PATIENTS' with patient card, insurance etc. The food we eat is to increase the Glucose (sugar) intake to sustain metabolic routine. From today, you can eat your favorite candies, pastry in moderation as you like. There is nothing harm in it. Sugar candies made up of jaggery is good for health. You should avoid 'powdered white sugar (India)' as it contains sulphur which is very harmful to your body.

From Illness to Wellness!!!

"SPICE" TASTE TREATMENT

To HEAL ASTHMA, Constipation, SINUS & other Respiratory Diseases etc. (LUNGS-NOSE-AIR PRANA SHAKTHI, Large Intestines)

The moment you taste a spicy food, It will transform into AIR prana shakthi to activate "LUNGS". Your NOSE-LUNGS will look alike, though varying in size. In similar terms, Large intestines and LUNGS are interrelated. If you've deficient **AIR** intake, then it will lead to constipation. In summary, you should understand the relation between NOSE-LUNGS & INTESTINES. Hence, those who're suffering from either constipation and/or ashtma ailments should take appropriate steps to increase the air intake thorugh the breathing techniques to heal the condition.

Also, as we discused your relation to emotions will cause disturbances. When you're sad, then your breathing will increase. The "SAD" state of emotion will discharge prana shakthi, and you'll feel the deficit as your cells will get tired. This could also be a reson for the sickness mentioned above. You should remember, each of your emotional state of mind haas its varying consequences at the organ level.

In summary, you should take enough quantity of taste in proportion in a daily meal as required by the individuals. You'll need to determine what you'll need to keep yourself healthy. After all, Nature is taking to you directly & not to your family Doctors.

From Illness to Wellness!!!

"BITTER" Tatste Treatment

To clear poison content in blood. The bitter taste is related to the FIRE. It will distribute FIRE prana shakthi throughout the BODY. The BITTER taste is related to the emotion of HAPPINESS. The color of tongue is an indication of HEART diseases. Hence, Doctor's ask you show the tongue for **'DIAGNOSIS'**. You must add BITTER tase to your daily intake. It will help you heal HEART related diseaes.

One more point…In ancient siddha medicines, Whenever there is a snake bite, saints will prescribe a bitter "CHIRIYA-Nangai" herbs to the patient. It tastes BITTER. This herb has 'FIRE' shakthi. This FIRE shakthi will induce HEART positively to eliminate poison in BLOOD. If there is a SNAKE BITE, neem leaves or bitter guard have ability to remove poison in **BLOOD.**

I've **HEARD** a story, which is a real one. A gardener was bitten by a SNAKE. He was absolutely al right for almost FOUR days, until his friend asked him what was the bit on the toes. He just looked at it, and the friend said..Perhaps, it looks like a **SNAKE** bite. Immediately, the gardner fell down unconscious and died. It has do with the FEAR, ANXIETY which has affected the kidneys. Hence, **DO NOT FEAR ANYTHING IN THE WORLD.** PLEASE do not fear anything. I am not saying you should avoid Doctors, take necessary emergency medication to prevent poison reaching the organs. Neeem leaves / bottle guard should be taken in regular dosage in your daily meal to boost your IMMUNE levels as you know it

From Illness to Wellness!!!

enhances FIRE shakthi. Indeed, whenever your tounge tastes BITTER, is an indication of NATURE removing poison in BLOOD.

In India there is a tradition, where some of the devotees will pierce their nose and tounge with spears. If you closely observe them, they will be chewing neem leaves and lemon. Do you know the reason why? There is an enormous loss of FIRE shakthi in the body, hence the heart rate (BP) will increase significantly. In order to restore FIRE shakthi, these devotees will chew neem leaves and lemon.

Hence, you should understand the lineage between Bitter taste to the following:
FIRE Shakthi-Temperature control glands-Tongue with the Emotions of Happines etc.
The one who understands this lineage is the one who can CURE DISEASES.

Your TONGUE IS A doctor and TASTE IS MEDICINE: Whenever your tongue demands for a specific taste, you should take appropriate food for it. FOR example. During pregnancy, women will ask for a SALT taste in mango. It's Nature's plan…she will demand variety of taste SALT, SUGAR, and SOUR, SPICE. You must provide a good meal during the pregnancy, as the foetus grows in the body, there is a lot of fire, air, land & prana shakthi required. Hence, in India they celebrate before the first child is born they host a festival with six variety of food to relish her taste buds with SALT, SOUR, BITTER etc. This festival is called 'SEEMANDHAM'. The ancient India

From Illness to Wellness!!!

had science in it with profound wisdom, which is being lost by the contemporary medicine. These are profound Natural healing methods, and liaising closely with the mother.Nature.

Nowadays, technology has improved with scans and tests. Your Doctors will advice you about the SUGAR levels in blood and request you to reduce SUGAR intake, defying NATURE's design and plan. Nature talks to you through taste buds. I request you to listen to it. You must appreciate women asking for variety of taste during her pregnancy period. This would help in the foetus development. If you suppress, lead to many complications in the CHILD birth & deficiencies. Hence, you've lost the natural process of DELIVERY. Why have you lost the ability to DELIVER a baby naturally. If animals can succeed in giving birth Naturally.

To summary, friends think about the taste intake these days. Your Doctors have adviced SUGAR isn't good for Diabetic, SALT isn't good for BP, tamrind isn't good for Arthritis so on and so forth. Then, what else to taste? It's a wrong notion. You've understood the ultimate DOCTOR functions through the TONGUE & heals through TASTE buds. There is no need to MESS up with the ultimate NATURE's system. Just be passionate to yourself, by listening to the wonders within. Eat when you're hungry, not angry! And provide enough attention to the the 300 Million cells within by giving good rest, where SLEEP functions as a Doctor.

From Illness to Wellness!!!

Excess consumption of Alcohol, Drugs, Tea, Coffee, non-alcoholic beverages

Have you noticed post your alchol consumption after a few hours, alcohol mixes with blood. It is poisonous, and LIVER your automechanic will try to eliminate poison in blood. As a result the LIVER is subjected to an extreme load of work depending on your consumption, eventually this will lead to LIVER damage. Hence, you should limit or avoid alchol consumption which is not good for health. Doctors do not indicate the drugs with extreme alcohol in it. It is poisonus, hence people who take regular medications, addicted to soda, alcoholic, non-alcoholic beverages will be affected. Tea, Coffee should be in moderation as it will stimulate your nervous system. The carbon is soda is dangerous. It should be thrown out of body, it is not something that you should consume!

From Illness to Wellness!!!

Process of Digestion
- **STEP 1** – Preliminary digestion in mouth
- **STEP 2** – Intestinal Digestion in intestines
- **STEP 3** – Transformation to nutrients in stomach using HCL which completes DIGESTIVE process

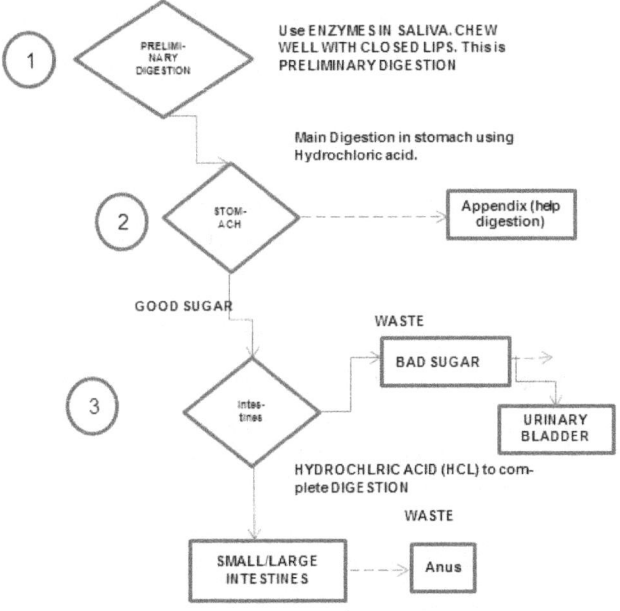

The **DIGESTIVE PROCESS INVOLVE** grinding the food, with preliminary digestion using SALIVA in mouth. The **SALIVA** will produce Enzymes for digestion. Secondly. The juice will pass through the long tube, the esophagus, into the stomach. Here, the food is mixed with powerful acids and other chemical enzymes such as pepsin. The stomach is designed

From Illness to Wellness!!!

to handle these powerful chemicals, which further digest your food. .

You've observed the fundamental diseases are originating in blood and the reasons as incomplet DIGESTION, leading to BAD cholesterol, sugar etc. These are residue due to lack of proper approach while eating. Ok. Then let me ask you a question?

INTESTINAL DIGESTION

After it leaves the stomach, partially digested food passes into the small intestines. Here, bile from the liver and digestive enzymes from the pancreas is added to the food mixture. These secretions of the liver and pancreas add more powerful chemicals to the human chemical factory to break down the food even more. These break down fats, starches, proteins and some sugars as well.

There are few rules as propounded by the ancient vedic scripturs:

From Illness to Wellness!!!

Vedic Rules of Eating Food

Rule # 1 – EAT FOOD ONLY WHEN YOU'RE HUNGRY. If you eat without hunger, it will transform in to BAD cholesterol & Sugar leading to all diseases. You're NOT a ROBO to be fed on-time, you're a organic unit. Hence. DO NOT follow the wall clock, instead listen to the digestive clock and your intestines. It will ask when the cells are hungry. You've to listen to the bio-rhythm. The fundamental REASONS for all DISEASES is due to the food that you EAT without being HUNGRY. Also, you should not keep the hunger long enough, since the body has prepared HCL acid to digest food in the intestines, it will send you alert messages of hunger in the form of blurb. You should start eating food slowly, consciously with all its due respect to satisfy the hunger of 300 Million cells.

I believe this is one of the reason, poor people are a lot healthier than the rich ones, those who have a laundry list of Diseases…have you observed? All these billionaires have a huge laundry list of diseases, since eating becomes a habit and you induldge.
Let us practice ways to accumulate wealth by health to have a richer heart, digestive, respiratory system. This is real WEALTHY. Please do remember this!

Rule # 2 – DO NOT COUNT # OF TIMES AND/OR OVEREAT or EAT in a hurry

From Illness to Wellness!!!

Eating THREE times a DAY is not in any constituition. Nature is a poetry, LOVE and it is not a constituitional framework. Each of your biology and metabolism varies depending on the work etc. Hence, you cannot generalize by saying EATING THREE TIMES a day is GOOD. The one who is working in the FIELD, a farmer will need food FIVE times a day, which is not true for a software Engineer who spends hours in front of a beloved, computer. Perhaps you may have to change your own LUNCH TIME. Or atleast you can follow few techniques to digest food properly.

As we discussed about HCL formed in stomach for DIGESTION. Now, say about 'X' ounce of HCL is formed to DIGEST 'Y' quantity of FOOD in stomach. If you've consumed "$Y+\alpha$" of food, then there is no adequate quanity of HCL to digest "α". Now, what happens to the "α" undigested food in stomach. Think about a food kept outide in room temperature for three days. It will spoil right. You're right. It will spoil in the stomach as well, leading to all sort of DISEASES. The spoiled food will lead to infections.

The same fundamentals apply to consumption of non-vegetarian food which are hard to DIGEST. The above phenonmen applies here as well. Please reduce your non-vegentarian food intake or become a pure Vegetarian. If you're busy, rather drink something like 9 grain shake naturally home made (India), instead of eating meal in a hurry, which would lead to excessive SUGAR/FAT into cholesterol/diabetes.

From Illness to Wellness!!!

Rule # 3 – CLOSE YOUR LIPS AND CHEW COMPLETELY TO MIX SALIVA IN FOOD.

You must eat slowly, chewing food adequately and mix SALIVA. Food that you eat without mixing SALIVA becomes a POISON. You've ENZYMES in your SALIVA. It helps in decomposing food completely. This is a priliminary step of digesting food in mouth, prior to the secondary process of digestion in the intestines. If you aren't digesting food through SALIVE in mouth, then food deposited in intestines will turn waste and poisonous. This is a basic science of eating food.

1. **Close your lips and chew food completely.** If your lips are open, then you will allow air inbetween the food & saliva, which will cause indigestion.

2. **DO NOT DRINK LIQUID WITH MEALS. DO NOT DRINK WATER 30 MINS BEFORE MEALS or 30 MINS AFTER MEAL.**

Remember AIR disturbs DIGESTIVE process in mouth, whilst WATER distrubs DIGESTIVE process in stomach. Hence, you should be aware of avoiding opening your lips while eating. And avoid water during meal.

In countries like **US, ITALY & JAPAN,** mostly they eat with closed lips by chewing food completely. I enjoy wathcing them eat slowly, consciously with profound wisdom. Unfortunately, India and many Eastern countries are losing its heritage due to ignorance. My observation is that people in INDIA,

From Illness to Wellness!!!

SINGARPORE, MALAYSIA..are eating in a hurry with open lips. Hence, there is an alarming increase in the number of DIABETIC's in the Eastern countries. If you flaunt the basic rules of Nature, you'll suffer. It is as simple as that!

Rule # 4 – FOCUS YOUR ATTENTION IN FOOD WHILE YOU'RE EATING in RELAXED MIND
You must focus your attention should be in food during the process of eating as negative emotions will hamper DIGESTIVE process. Someone asked a YOGI, "Please tell me ways to protect us from DISEASES" and yogi responded by saying:

"You should EAT, while you EAT"
And the disciple responded, Guru,…please explain.

"You should EAT, while you EAT" which means you should really EAT with BODY, MIND AND SPIRIT. You should remember your 300Million Cells as your children asking for food in hunger. Once you get the sensations of HUNGER, feel thankful to be alive, feel the food, prepare the heart and spirit and then EAT it in the state of meditation."

Atleast you should be prepared to focus your attention, thoughts in food while eating, be concious that you're eating food in "moderation" for wellness and it is a medicine. Be responsible, as you're not eating for sensual gratification alone. It should be be moderation as discussed before, realize the organs inside the body and 300 Million cells eating food, perhaps this is the reason why ancient system claims

From Illness to Wellness!!!

a Goddess 'Shakthi' with thousand eyes. It is a metaphor for the cells in the body, which has its intelligence. You should thank the ones who have prepared the food in family or restaurant; You must auto-suggest in mind that *'FOOD that I am taking will be digested & transformed to Blood, and a food for all organs. It is the ultimate medicine for all diseases'*

Saint Maharishi Vethathiri has said:
"You can see the communal integrity of the whole WHOLE WORLD in a handful of FOOD"
What a beautiful statement...! and he started explaining in one of the sessions. The paddy or wheat is cultivated by farmers, grains are cleansed by the factories and packaged by retail units for distribution. Now, your spouse, or mom has cooked a wonderful meal for you, with the required spices to relish your taste buds isn't? You should thank them all for their efforts.Above all, Nature has graciously offered it through the FIVE ELEMENTS. Thank Nature for all of it.

To summarize, Eating is a social responsbility to keep yourself healthy to lead a happy life. On the contrary, if you are diverted by the process of thinking in MIND, then you're are subjected to the emotions. These emotions will result in 'poisoning' food. In the process of thinking you'll activate BRAIN cells through the **VEGAS** nerves. These nerves will respond to the stimuli. For example. If you are thinking about your business, work or relationships while eating food, your VEGAS will instruct BRAIN

From Illness to Wellness!!!

cells to react. This may result in positive or negative response, instead of focusing your cells on DIGESTION. Your inner mechanism will be interrupted by the sudden deviation caused by the VEGAS nerves. It's like you have applied a sudden brake, haling your drive on a **I-101** high way. Your DIGESTIVE system is disturbed by your act of thinking while eating.

I'll teach you a simple meditation technique:
Let's practice this medication technique at your dinning table at convenient schedule. you should spare atleast **TEN** mintues for a healthy life.

 Practice this in the morning meditation

Start off with the following statement:
"LET THE DIVINE ENERGY HEAL ME, GUIDE ME AND PROTECT ME."
My body is made up of CELLS, visualize cells in MIND, and then say.;"My cells are relaxed, healthy and peaceful" I'll be aware while taking FOOD to nourish my cells. Relax, Relax, Relax. Relax your cells. Then focus your attention on the foot:

"Let the blood circulation, heat circulation, air circulation & magnetic energy circulation be streamlined. Relax, relax, relax"

REPEAT it internally in every part of your body starting from., foot, legs, knees, thighs, lower abdomen, stomach. Now, internal organs-stomach, liver, gall bladder, spleen, kidney, lungs, heart, throat,

From Illness to Wellness!!!

eyes, ears, nose, chin, shoulders, hands and brain (repeat the above statement in every organ).

 Relax your body, mind

You can practice a simplified version of the above medication once for 2-3 minutes prior to eating food to remain AWARE. ATLEAST state that "YOUR 200 Million cells are GOING to EAT". You can start with thanking everyone, and remember your organs are nourished by the food, which is the ultimate medicine. Repeat the statement below holding a handful of food (you should feel the food), three times and then proceed to eating FOOD.

'FOOD that I am going to eat will be digested & transformed to Blood, and a food for all organs. It is the ultimate medicine for all diseases. Let the DIVINE energy heal me, guide me and protect me'

Friends, In summary, I request you all to lead a simple, happy, healthy & prosperous life. There is no need to be worried about one-hundred & one things. Your busienss partner's can wait until you complete a meal, as the internal business partner's are there to help you. Your emotions are related to the organs, which will cause an impact in the system. Your TASTE buds is an alert system to help you. Follow your natural rhythm, there is no BETTER HEALER THAN YOUR NATURE. STAY TUNED TO NATURE. MEDITATION AND GOOD FOOD PRACTICES in simple and profound techniques of healing.

From Illness to Wellness!!!

Rule # 5 – CHEW YOUR FOOD BY USING TEETH.

DIGESTION BEGINS IN THE MOUTH
Chew your food at least 20 times for healthy digestion. Digestion begins in the mouth with chewing. Chewing mechanically breaks down food, and is very important. This is why bolting your food, or not chewing thoroughly, is a very bad habit and always leads to malnutrition. Only the mouth has teeth to mechanically tear apart the food.

In addition, chewing breaks down the food chemically. Chemicals in your saliva called amylase enzymes break down starches and other food components right in the mouth. Many people do not realize that some food components including some vitamins and minerals, sugars and others, can be absorbed directly from the mouth into the body.

Chewing each bite at least two dozen times or so is most helpful for good health. It may feel odd at first, but it quickly becomes a healthful habit. Chewing your food at least two dozen times each bite is also a simple and very healthful way to eat less and lose weight. Everyone else will be on their second or third portion and you will still be on your first portion. If you chew your food two dozen times, you will also feel full a lot faster.

If you absolutely cannot chew food thoroughly for some reason, then blend, puree or juice the food in a blender, food processor or juicer. This is not as good

From Illness to Wellness!!!

as chewing. However, it is much better than swallowing food without proper chewing. If you're eating food without proper chewing, then the workload of stomach will increase. The quantity of required HCL will be less to digest the excess food, since you've not used the preliminary digestion in mouth by chewing it properly. End result is that you'll have undigested food in stomach resulting in increased tummy, body weight etc. If you want to lose excess weight, chew your food completely. The rule is that you should chew at least 15-20 times & DO NOT DRINK FLUIDS. If you're terribly thirsty, drink ¼ glass of water only if it absolutely necessary.

DO NOT FOLLOW YOUR DOCTORS ADVICE
Your Doctors will advise you to take tablets post your meal. Now, you will take medications after a heavy meal, and DRINK lots of water. What happens?
Did you know the water that you drink will interrupt your digestion in stomach; half of your food will go undigested leading to increasing your diseases. Instead of controlling your disease through allopathic medications, it has led to another disease. You'd have increased SUGAR, Cholesterol, and Indigestion etc. This is how your headache created by Doctors will turn into stomach ache and many more to follow. If you're in a situation to take medications, then wait thirty minutes post meal and take it.

ULCER

From Illness to Wellness!!!

The main reason for Ulcer is due to eating **FOOD ON-TIME**, not while you're really hungry. The excess undigested food that is already there in stomach will be stagnated; you'll add up another sitting of meal, which would cause over stacked.

Rule # 6 – Do not Eat while watching TV, mobile, DVD, Tele serials, Internet, ipad, ipod, laptop etc. Avoid eating out frequently
You should avoid anything that will distract your focus on food. You should give some respect to the 300 Million cells asking for food. And you should find the holistic unity of FIVE ELEMENTS (Pancha Boothas are linked to your body; hence you should not eat watching TV. If you do so, then the entire focus will be on TV, leading to emotional imbalance. This will impact digestion as you know the DIGESTIVE process is interrupted by the glands that secrete when you're worried or extremely happy talking to your girlfriend or worried fighting with your wife etc. If you're eating with your spouse or girl-friend, just enjoy the meal totally without any gossip.

You're organically linked with the Universe, feel blessed and eat every bit of food with a social responsibility. You got to remember your 300Million children (cells) asking for food. If you treat them well, they will keep you healthy without disease. Wouldn't you agree your children can influence the moods? You're happy only if they are happy. They can rattle your happiness isn't? So. Treat your children with respect & love both your progeny outside & inside the body. There is nothing called a "working meal"…If you continue working meal. You'll soon be

From Illness to Wellness!!!

diagnosed for Diabetes, Cholesterol etc. Would you want a working meal or a happy meal? Think for a moment.

Rule # 7 DO NOT read books or board room discussions while eating meal.
Apparently, your lunch time seems to be the gossip time at work, when you throw negativity about others, it will impact you first. Remember, it will hamper the Digestive process. Your mood fluctuations will secrete few glands that will hamper the Digestive process. You know if you talk, the AIR entering your mouth will hamper the preliminary DIGESTIVE process in mouth. DO NOT TALK while eating at least from now on. Do not talk business over a dining table. If you've something to talk urgently, talk in between the meal, not while having food in mouth. I have observed in many restaurants, the time for dinner is the best time to express your love to others!!! What about love for food. The objectives are lost; as a result defying LAWS of NATURE will result in diseases later on. You can propose your love after you have a good meal. She will appreciate your patience!

I have heard someone saying…Potato is not good, Onion is not good, Brinjal or coconut etc. If you keep on listening to such things, you'll never be able to eat anything .Instead. Follow a good meal practices with the rules of Vedic scriptures. You'll be able to heal yourself and lead a healthy life. You should avoid white-sugar which has poisonous chemical 'Sulphur' which will impact your digestive track.

From Illness to Wellness!!!

You must avoid processed food, smoking, or alcohol habits if you have any. The best posture for eating food is in a sitting posture as in ancient wisdom. You've be in a sitting posture not on a chair, likely with folded legs. This will enhance the blood circulation through the upper organs in your body, above hip. Your essential organs such as Kidney, Pancreas, Liver, Brain, Eyes and Ears are above the hip. Otherwise, if you always keep your legs down, your blood circulation will be towards the lower organs of the body. This will reduce your IMMUNE levels. The one who sits in the Suk asana posture with folded legs will be able to conserve more energy. One of the main reasons of knee joint problems is mainly due to sitting in chairs mostly with legs down. If you try sitting with folded legs at least few times, it will heal.

The food prepared at home has its' own taste & emotions. The food prepared in restaurants with artificial flavors, taste will addict your sense-tongue. Moreover, the emotions of the cook will impact overall. If you're taking a homemade food, the feel of food will be good as the emotions of the spouse, or mom will impact the food positively or negatively. I've observed a Guru identifying the emotions in a house based on the taste of food….

A saint said…to the disciple…

"Disciple, Nanda…I can see someone is sick and unhealthy today…"

How do you Swami? As the disciple exclaimed

From Illness to Wellness!!!

I can feel the sad vegetables…you seem to be affecting the atmosphere with your emotions. Be happy and cook a meal that is healthy, natural with lots of vegetables, sprouts for your family!!!

Rule # 6 – A) **DO NOT BATHE FOR TWO HOURS POST heavy MEAL,**

B) **DO NOT EAT heavy MEAL FOR 45 MINS POST YOU BATHE.**

Let's analyze what happnes while you bathe. YOUR BODY temperature is moderated by **'Triple Warmer'** which manages your body temperature to 37 Degree Centigrade. If you take a warm bath or a cold bath, your Triple warmer will take some time to re adjust your 37Degree C.

Hence, it will impact the DIGESTIVE system, when the gland is active. YOU MUST AVOID TAKING BATH RIGHT AFTER A GOOD MEAL. Give it some time post meal for two hours interval. In similar terms, you should not bathe and take food right after. There should be a minimal interval of 45 mins to get back to normal. You might have different work routine, etc. However, you cannot make an excuse for all these trivial reasons as your BODY system follows a simple rhythm. I believe even animals are sensitive to Nature as they are completely aligned, except human beings who have travelled far off from the

From Illness to Wellness!!!

Nature. It's imaginary, you should get back to Nature to heal yourself.

Rule # 7 – Know your belching or burbing symptoms ("yeppam")

  A) **Burbing before eating food**

As we discussed when you're hungry, your system will produce HCL acid in stomach for digestion. Your burbing or belching is an indication of your system being hungry. You'll feel the sensation of hunger. Hence. You'll need to eat at that time. If you are unable to eat good meal, then take some fruits atleast. However. If you're travelling or something without being able to eat, you should drink water to liquidate the acid. Otherwise, this will lead to ulcer.

  B) **Burbing after eating food. This is a good sign of digestion.**

There is a window opening from stomach to intestines. The window at the bottom of stomach wills it completes digestion. It's interesting to study nature's design; burbing is due to the air coming in to the stomach. The noise of air filling in stomach, which enters from the upper opening of stomach, is burbing.

YOU MUST OBSERVE THESE SYMPTOMS:

1. DO NOT EAT FOOD WITHOUT HUNGER

From Illness to Wellness!!!

2. STOP EATING FOOD AFTER THE FIRST BURP, WHICH IS AN INDICATION OF DIGESTED FOOD IN STOMACH, PASSED ON TO THE INTESTINES. FURTHER, THE AIR IS TAKEN IN TO THE STOMACH FROM THE WINDOW OPENING.

If you feel hungry, eat again.
Rule # 8 – WOMEN SHOULD TAKE CARE OF EATING HEALTY WITH CARE IN MODERATION

Maharishi Vethathiri has said:
'WOMEN ARE BORN ENLIGHTENED. There is no need for them to be enlightened'.
Nature has made her unique with the ability to re-produce. This is part of Nature's intrinsic design. A mom's emotional changes will impact the fetus in pregnancy. Hence, it is mandatory to allow your spouse to support her needs & take good care of her. Especially, her body changes in menstrual cycle, it goes through a significant biological process.

From Illness to Wellness!!!

Rule # 9 – TRY EVERY MEAL WITH GOOD SIX TASTES IN MODERATION
REMEMEBER this picture.

Sweet, Sour, Salty, Bitter, Pungent, and Astringent. While the first four tastes are probably recognizable, the last two may not seem familiar. Pungent taste is hot and spicy as found in a chili pepper, while Astringent taste is dry and light as found in popcorn.

Include all 6 Tastes in each meal

The SIX tastes us a user-friendly guide map for how to nourish ourselves. Instead of looking at nutritional labels for X amount of protein or Y amount of carbohydrates, the 6 Tastes naturally guide us towards our body's nutritional needs. Each taste feeds our mind, body, senses, and spirit in its own unique way. From a modern nutritional perspective, the SIX Tastes satisfy each of the major dietary building blocks. Sweet foods, for example, are rich in fats, proteins, carbohydrates, and water, whereas Bitter and Astringent foods are high in vitamins and minerals.

From Illness to Wellness!!!

The brain sends the body signals when it requires energy in the form of food. By incorporating all 6 Tastes into each meal, we ensure that these signals are adequately met, thus avoiding food cravings or the over-consumption of certain foods...Including the 6 tastes in each meal doesn't need to be a daunting task. Adding a squeeze of lemon to cooked dishes, for example, can quickly satisfy the Sour taste, while adding a side salad will fulfill the Bitter and Astringent tastes.

2) Allow your unique constitution to determine the proportion of tastes you eat: The body naturally desires tastes that balance its doshic makeup and shuns tastes of an aggravating nature. In this sense, things are made pretty easy for us: If we simply follow our natural inclinations, we are led to the proper foods. Vata individuals, for example, are naturally drawn to moist, grounding foods, while Kapha individuals favor light, drying foods.

Our ancient Indian wisdom in Ayurveda nutrition recommends includes all 6 tastes in each meal, while favoring those tastes that bring greater balance to your particular constitution. A Pitta individual, for example, will favor cooling foods and spices such as dark leafy greens and fennel, which are high in Bitter and Astringent tastes, while requiring a smaller quantity of the Pungent taste.

SWEET
Sweet taste results from the combination of Water and Earth and is heavy, moist, and cooling by na-

From Illness to Wellness!!!

ture. In the West, sugary foods are most commonly associated with this taste. Sweet taste is also found in milk and milk products (like butter, ghee, and cream), most grains (especially wheat, rice, and barley), many legumes (like beans and lentils), sweet fruits (such as bananas and mangos), and certain cooked vegetables (such as carrots, sweet potatoes, and beets).

Sweet taste naturally increases bulk, moisture, and weight in the body. For this reason, it is excellent for building the body's seven vital tissues (called *dhatus*) of plasma, blood, fat, muscles, bones, marrow, and reproductive fluids. Sweet taste also increases saliva, soothes mucous membranes and burning sensations, relieves thirst, and has beneficial effects on the skin, hair, and voice.

SOUR
Sour Taste is composed of Earth and Fire and is hot, light, and moist by nature. It is commonly found in citrus fruits (such as lemon and limes), sour milk products (like yogurt, cheese, and sour cream), and fermented substances (including wine, vinegar, pickles, sauerkraut, and soy sauce). Used in moderation, Sour taste stimulates digestion, helps circulation and elimination, energizes the body, strengthens the heart, relieves thirst, maintains acidity, sharpens the senses, and helps extract minerals such as iron from food. It also nourishes all the vital tissues (dhatus) except the reproductive tissues (the exception being yogurt,

From Illness to Wellness!!!

which nourishes all the tissues).

SALTY
Salty taste is composed of Fire and Water and is hot, heavy, and moist by nature. It is found in any salt (such as sea salt and rock salt), sea vegetables (like seaweed and kelp), and foods to which large amounts of salt are added (like nuts, chips, and pickles). Due to its drying quality in the mouth, it may seem counterintuitive to think of Salty taste as moistening. The element of Water in its composition, however, relates to its water retaining quality. Salty taste falls somewhere between Sweet and Sour tastes with regard to its heavy and moist qualities.

In moderation, Salty taste improves the flavor of food, improves digestion, lubricates tissues, liquefies mucous, maintains mineral balance, aids in the elimination of wastes, and calms the nerves. Due to its tendency to attract water, it also improves the radiance of the skin and promotes overall growth in the body.

PUNGENT
Pungent taste derives from the elements of Fire and Air and is hot, dry, and light. It is the hottest of all the 6 Tastes and is found in certain vegetables (such as chili peppers, garlic, and onions), and in spices (like black pepper, ginger, and cayenne). In small amounts, Pungent taste stimulates digestion, clears the sinuses, promotes sweating and detoxification, dispels gas, aids circulation, im-

From Illness to Wellness!!!

proves metabolism, and relieves muscle pain.

BITTER
Bitter taste is composed of Air and Ether and is light, cooling, and dry by nature. It is found in green leafy vegetables (such as spinach, kale, and green cabbage), other vegetables (including zucchini and eggplant), herbs and spices (like turmeric, fenugreek, and dandelion root), coffee, tea, and certain fruits (such as grapefruits, olives, and bitter melon). While Bitter taste is often not appealing alone, it stimulates the appetite and helps bring out the flavor of the other tastes. Bitter taste is a powerful detoxifying agent, and has antibiotic, anti-parasitic, and antiseptic qualities. It is also helpful in reducing weight, water retention, skin rashes, fever, burning sensations and nausea

ASTRINGENT

Astringent taste results from the combination of Air and Earth and is dry, cooling, and heavy by nature. It is the least common of all the 6 Tastes and can be found in legumes (such as beans and lentils), fruits (including cranberries, pomegranates, pears, and dried fruit), vegetables (such as, broccoli, cauliflower, artichoke, asparagus and turnip), grains (such as rye, buckwheat, and quinoa), spices and herbs (including turmeric and marjoram), coffee, and tea. Astringent taste is not as cold as Bitter taste but has a greater cooling effect on the body than Sweet taste.

From Illness to Wellness!!!

Astringent taste is classified more in relation to its effect on the tongue than its actual taste. It creates a puckering sensation in the mouth (such as cranberries) or a dry, chalky feeling (such as many beans). Foods like broccoli or cauliflower have a mildly Astringent taste that is less detectable. Dry foods such as crackers and chips, most raw vegetables, and the skins of fruits also have Astringent qualities.

HOW MUCH TASTE SHOULD I TAKE? It depends on individual to individual; hence use your inner discretion while eating your meal. In ancient wisdom of India, they had served a small quantity of SWEET before you start your meal. This will stimulate YOUR DIGESTIVE SYSTEM. As discussed earlier, TASTE as much as you can. You'll get PRANA shakthi through TASTE and food that you consume. Only tongue can TASTE and not your stomach, hence relish your food in moderation.

ADDICTIONS TO FOOD

Mostly addictions to food are due to the artificial flavors and packaged foods. When food is commercialized, you get addicted. These companies add chemicals to boost taste artificially such as Biscuits, Cool drinks, savories. Hence, if you're taking artificial packaged chips, savories etc…Then the Natural medicine will not work and the entire program will be a waste of time.

You must avoid carbonated drinks, and artificial packaged food. The basic fundamentals of taste that

From Illness to Wellness!!!

we are discussing here is Natural taste of your tongue to enjoy the natural taste available in food. This artificial chemical flavored food such as noodles, food cooked in restaurants and harmful. They will create an imbalance and false sensations for pleasure. You'll be addicted to the false sensations which you might think as taste. DO NOT EAT packaged food or eating out in the restaurants should be avoided for your healthy life. It's simple and profound if you follow. For elders without tooth. Prefer a liquefied diet, or perhaps you can grind food before serving.

Vedic Methods of Water Purification

DO NOT BOIL AND/OR FILTER WATER Water ($H20$). If you're boiling water to kill germs. What about germs in air. You are inhaling 11,500 Liters of air every day. Now, would you heat air before you inhale? As we discussed about germs in the earlier chapters, you're aware about the INCREDIBLE FOUR IMMUNE system that will fight the germs. There is no need to boil water. Water consists of Prana shakthi and germs. If you boil, you exhaust both of them. You're losing vitamins, minerals, prana shakthi by boiling water. Boiled water loses all its vitamins, minerals and prana shakthi that you'll need for blood constituents. It helps you build immune naturally. I will explain a simple technique to witness this all by you.

Take a small bowl of boiled water…once it comes to the room temperature, let a fish. You'll be surprised

From Illness to Wellness!!!

to see the fish dying. Even a fish cannot survive in the boiled water. What you're drinking is of no use to the system. There are no vitamins, minerals to nourishing you from the water that you're drinking.

However, in an emergency period such as flood...and other major calamities, there is a possibility that water is contaminated with dead animals, human beings. It is essential to filter, boil during this time but not as a general practice. If you're using a water filter, then rest assured, you are throwing away minerals, vitamins deposited in the filter. Hence, you'll be deficient of these vitamins, minerals in Blood. Eventually you'll lose the IMMUNE system. Have you noticed Easterner's those are travelling abroad do not get sick by drinking water? Mostly Westerner's, those who travel to East fall sick next day. This is due to the variation in the immune levels, and the Immunity was higher in those days in East, where there was no water filter and body naturally produced IMMUNITY, whilst the minerals, vitamins were available for the BLOOD to build a solid body with good IMMUNE system. All packaged bottled water separates minerals, vitamins, hence there is no value add to the blood by drinking such low grade Water. The **'Anti-Scale Dosing'** machine used in factories for water purification will filter all essential minerals. Hence, you'll be devoid of nutrients with a low IMMUNE system.

1. **Did you know a clay pot made in those days is an excellent water purifier?** It will filter water, and it will add 'LAND' shakthi to water.

From Illness to Wellness!!!

2. **Filter water with soft white cotton cloth. Cotton cloth will absorb bacteria, virus in water.**
3. **Banana skin -** Use Banana skin in the clay pot filled with water. This will absorb virus, bacteria. However, you should take necessary care not to store Banana skin in the pot beyond thirty minutes.
4. **Use Copper made pot to store water for 2-5 hours will energize water & also removes virus/bacteria - Did** you know using Cu will purify water? Or perhaps you can drop Copper made coins in to the mud pot. If you observe Hindu scriptures, you would have noticed Saints carrying a small kettle made of copper. If a demon disturbs, they will give a bane with the water in the copper. This is just a story to indicate the power of water stored in Copper. It energizes you positively.

5. A simple test to check if you've DISEASES in the body. Try a simple method of self-test. If you're getting running nose/FLUM due to a change in drinking normal water, which indicates your body is trying to assimilate nutrients that you've not supplied till date. Hence, it will start its process of extracting waste in your body to eliminate it via FLUM, SINUS, and running nose as discussed.
6. **How much quantity of water should I drink?** Your water consumption cannot be generalized as 1-2 or 3-4 Liters/day. It depends on various factors from person to person depending on the age, work, climate and surrounding atmosphere

From Illness to Wellness!!!

etc. A simple rule of thumb is to drink water when you're thirsty. If you're forcing yourself to drink water without being thirsty, you'll eventually end up in Kidney problems. If you're ignoring your thirst, your body cells will extract water from the organs, leading to a different sort of problems. So. Bottom line, drink when you're thirsty. Follow your body discipline.

7. **Eat WATER** – This indicates you should take sip by sip and taste it mixing with you SALIVA. This will help you absorb minerals from water. It has all six tastes in it. Drink adequate quantity of water as required post you urinate. A small test to determine your drinking water safety. Test it by dropping a fish in to a bowl of drinking water & observe for an hour, it if is good and has enough prana shakthi, then its drinkable.

AIR

DID YOU KNOW YOU INHALE 8 LITRE AIR/MIN? Only human beings seem to have enclosed him with in a house, whilst the entire Universe is available to him to enjoy. Most of the homes remain with closed windows. How do you feel energized, and most you sleep with all windows closed?

AIR contains Oxygen, Nitrogen, and Hydrogen & Prana shakthi. It will be mixed with blood to distribute it to the respective cell functions / organs. If you remember the train and the station analogy, your blood will carry nutrients absorbed from air and distribute it to the organs, which are like railway station.

From Illness to Wellness!!!

The nutrient exchange will happen, and the waste is sent back to the blood. From blood to nostrils, where you'd exhale. Let us analyze the step by step process. It is important to understand the process of breathing.

Process of Breathing

- **STEP 1** – Preliminary filteration of Air in the Nostrils
- **STEP 2** – Intestinal Digestion in intestines
- **STEP 3** – Transformation to nutrients in stomach using HCL which completes DIGESTIVE process

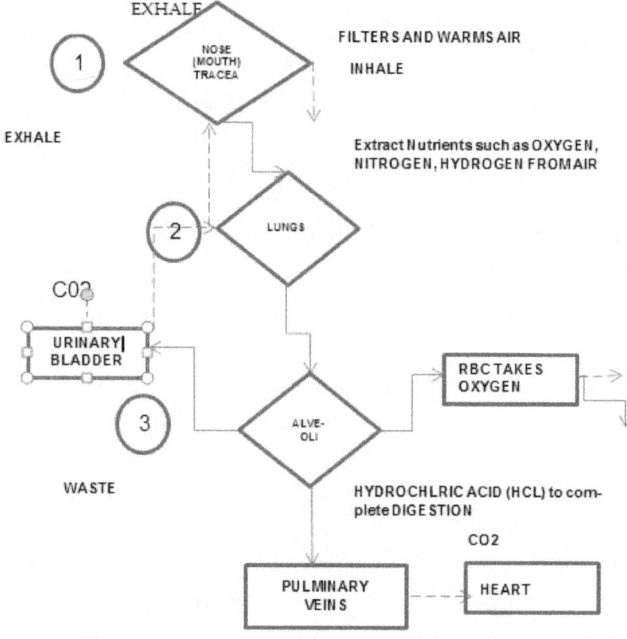

What Happens When You Breathe?

From Illness to Wellness!!!

Breathing In (Inhalation): When you breathe in, or inhale, your diaphragm contracts (tightens) and moves downward. This increases the space in your chest cavity, into which your lungs expand. The intercostal muscles between your ribs also help enlarge the chest cavity. They contract to pull your rib cage both upward and outward when you inhale.

As your lungs expand, air is sucked in through your nose or mouth. The air travels down your windpipe and into your lungs. After passing through your bronchial tubes, the air finally reaches and enters the alveoli (air sacs).

Through the very thin walls of the alveoli, oxygen from the air passes to the surrounding capillaries (blood vessels). A red blood cell protein called hemoglobin (HEE-muh-glow-bin) helps move oxygen from the air sacs to the blood. At the same time, carbon dioxide moves from the capillaries into the air sacs. The gas has traveled in the bloodstream from the right side of the heart through the pulmonary artery.

Oxygen-rich blood from the lungs is carried through a network of capillaries to the pulmonary vein. This vein delivers the oxygen-rich blood to the left side of the heart. The left side of the heart pumps the blood to the rest of the body. There, the oxygen in the blood moves from blood vessels into surrounding tissues.

Breathing Out (Exhalation): When you breathe out, or exhale, your diaphragm relaxes and moves upward into the chest cavity. The intercostal

From Illness to Wellness!!!

muscles between the ribs also relax to reduce the space in the chest cavity. As the space in the chest cavity gets smaller, air rich in carbon dioxide is forced out of your lungs and windpipe, and then out of your nose or mouth.

Breathing out requires no effort from your body unless you have a lung disease or are doing physical activity. When you're physically active, your abdominal muscles contract and push your diaphragm against your lungs even more than usual. This rapidly pushes air out of your lungs.

 Avoid mosquito repellants which is dangerous to your respiratory system

STOP USING ANY MEDICATION FOR SLEEP. THIS WILL AFFECT YOUR ORGANS IN THE LONGER RUN. A simple meditation will help you relax your mind and body. It will help you to limit your thinking process, when it is not required. If you're able to relax a few minutes before you sleep or perhaps the best method is to lie down and relax every organ. Slowly auto suggests "My cells are relaxed, I am going to sleep" repeat it from the toes to the head every organ and finally suggest that you're going to sleep. A good sleep will heal you as it does the repair of cells.

From Illness to Wellness!!!

🚫 ALARM WILL ABRUPTLY WAKE UP YOU. YOU SHOULD NOT DO THAT AS IT WILL INDUCE TENSION IN THE BODY.

🚫 If you go to sleep post watching a movie…your MIND will not rest peacefully. It will induce thinking process.. If you are suffering from sleepless disorder, we have a technique in the acupressure (DU-20). Your body has 72,000 Nerves. A head massage is good to streamline magnetic flow blockages.

🚫 AVOID too much of TEA/COFFEE, SMOKING which will cause sleeping disorder. You can DRINK TEA/COFFEE depending on the country..If you're in a cold country it is good to warm up drinking TEA/COFFEE in moderation, however it should be restricted to the place where it is cultivated.

Eat fruits, vegetables etc. available in the respective state…There is no need to pay a very high premium to eat a Kashmir apple.. There is no need to pay "Oats" in countries like India where wheat based products are available aplenty.

✓ I'll teach you a simple meditation to help you sleep well. HimmmmM (pronounced as "himmmm") in "CHIN" mudra and keep breathing in and breath

From Illness to Wellness!!!

out with the "himmmmm" sound. Do it for 50 times, you'll get good sleep.

SLEEPING POSTURE-NORTH-SOUTH POLE

Your body is organically linked with the Universe, and the magnetic circuit. Your body can be classified as 'ABOVE NAVEL' & 'BELOW NAVEL'. There will be disturbances in the magnetic circuit, if the flow is interrupted then it will reduce your quality of sleep, it will cause interruption in the blood circulation, magnetic circulation leading to diseases.

It is BEST if your head is rested "SOUTH" The magnetic N-S will attract, and the N-N deflect. Similarly, your head rested in "NORTH"…it will cause magnetic disturbances. Hence. Vasthu shastra indicates resting your HEAD facing 'SOUTH' pole is the BEST to enable the magnetic circuit flow between your body and the earth 'NORTH' pole.

WORK – YOGA SADHANA

It is essential to maintain an active life style for good & healthy heart. A daily practice is required to keep yourself healthy. I recommend daily routine with YOGA exercies with meditation. This routine will energize you…

In the Ashtanga ("eight limbs") Yoga of Patanjali, the stage of meditation preceding dhyāna is called dharana. In Dhyana, the meditator is not conscious of the act of meditation (i.e. is not aware

From Illness to Wellness!!!

that s/he is meditating) but is only aware that s/he exists (consciousness of being), and aware of the object of meditation. Dhyana is distinct from Dharana in that the meditator becomes one with the object of meditation. This means that the meditator although aware of the object through meditation detaches him/erself from its existence in the physical world.

Much like meditation focused on the breath Dhyana is rooted in the concentration of not being concentrated. Ultimately Dhyana leads to the final stage of Yoga, Samādhi. He/she is then able to maintain this oneness for 144 inhalations and expiration.

Dhyana, practiced together with Dharana and Samādhi constitutes the Samyama. Samyama's goal is to fully detach the mind from its physical world bindings. This aids the Yogis in reaching an enlightenment where a self or spirit is truly acknowledged, and made aware of. Samyama also can lead to one's accomplishment of repelling the human need for objects putting the Yogis in a state of self-satisfaction.

The Dhyana Yoga system is specifically described by Sri Krishna in chapter 6 of the Bhagavad Gita, wherein He explains the many different Yoga systems to His friend and disciple, Arjuna. In fact, Lord Shankar described 108 different ways to do Dhyana to Mata Parvati.

From Illness to Wellness!!!

In Hinduism, dhyāna is considered to be an instrument to gain self-knowledge, separating māyā from reality to help attain the ultimate goal of mokṣa. Depictions of Hindu yogis performing dhyāna are found in ancient texts and in statues and frescoes of ancient Indian temples.

The Bhagavad Gītā, thought to have been written some time between 400 and 100 BC, talks of four branches of yoga:

- Karma Yoga: The yoga of action in the world
- Jnāna yoga: The yoga of Wisdom and intellectual endeavor
- Bhakti Yoga: The yoga of devotion to God
- Dhyāna Yoga: The yoga of meditation

Dhyāna in Rāja Yoga is also found in Patañjali's Yoga Sūtras. Practiced together with dhāraṇā and samādhi it constitutes the saṃyama.

For example, in the Jangama Dhyāna technique, the meditator concentrates the mind and sight between the eyebrows. According to Patañjali, this is one method of achieving the initial concentration (dhāraṇā: Yoga Sutras, III: 1) necessary for the mind to become introverted in meditation (dhyāna: Yoga Sutras, III: 2). In deeper practice of the technique, the mind concentrated between the eyebrows begins to automatically lose all location and focus on the watching itself. Eventually, the meditator experiences only the consciousness of existence and achieves self

From Illness to Wellness!!!

realization. Swami Vivekananda describes the process in the following way:

When the mind has been trained to remain fixed on a certain internal or external location, there comes to it the power of flowing in an unbroken current, as it were, towards that point. This state is called dhyana. When one has so intensified the power of dhyana as to be able to reject the external part of perception and remain meditating only on the internal part, the meaning, that state is called Samadhi.[5]

The **Discipline of Yoga** comprises of the following:

1. IMAYAM – Learning CAUSE and Effect system of Nature. Awareness about BODY, MIND, INTELLECT & ATMA (SOUL)
2. NIYAMAM – ELIMINATE harmful effects by practicing good actions that will yield good results.
3. ASANA – Excercises designed unique for the muscles and bones
4. PRANAYAMA – Streamlining your breathing pattern to increase Prana shakthi
5. PRAKTHIYAKARA – Realization of the sense and awareness while using the five senses …EAR, NOSE, TASTE, EYES, TOUCH & THINKING. It is your responsibility to use senses within limits. I f you exceed limits, each of these senses will be impacted.
6. DHARANA – Focusing your attention at a specific thought…analysis etc

From Illness to Wellness!!!

7. DHYANA – Dhyana is meditation, which is doing nothing.
8. SAMADHI – A deep state of alignment with the eternal consciousness.

If you understand the first two points in the DISCIPLINE OF YOGA…It is Vedic Healing. Awareness to do it right. Our Vedic Healing includes Achara, Anushtana, which means teaching you good habits and principles to practice for life-time. You can approach SIMPLIFIED KUNDALINI YOGA (SKY) or any other Yoga practices which is a profound method with exercies, acupressure and kundalini meditation. The kaya kalpa yoga taught here is very profound, which includes transmutation of the sexual vital fluid to prana shakthi to rejuvenate your body, mind and soul.

MIND-INTELLECT

"The Other End of Mind is GOD" – Maharishi Vethathiri…The core of mind is consciounss and the surface is conditioned. Your mind can be aligned to the eternal consciousness or just let go in the sensual pleasures. The habits form a prime reaosns, genetics which are form your baseline personality. If you would like to suceed in life in transcending conditioning, Yoga sadhana is the way to be aligned with the INTELLECT.

You should take decisions in aligment with the INTELLECT in uinson with the DIVINE JUSTICE. The INNER consciuosness will always reveal TRUTH,

From Illness to Wellness!!!

If you miss the truth, then you'll fall in to the vicious circle of repeating mistakes and results. Whenever you're taking decisions, make sure the results will not harm you, family or others, It should be in unison with the Divine Justice.

Your thoughts are your life. Ignore and DO NOT give any importance to the negative thoughts. Just observe, be aware, it will vanish. You should treat them like unwanted guests. It will disappear. If you want to know more about MIND... You can approach SKY (Vethathiri Maharishi) centers worldwide.

You've to stream line the following FIVE factors discussed throughout the book
     FOOD, AIR, WATER, REST & WORK.
If you practice this therapy regularly. You'll be healed within a year. The only exception is if you've gone through any organ transplant, your system will treat it as a foreign object. Hence you should not stop medications. Follow your doctor's advice. For all others. You should be able to completely stop medicines, and start living your life. The irony is that in Vedic Healing, there are no rules to follow. Perhaps the only rule is to eat when you're hungry with simple procedures to observe.

HOLISTIC UNITY OF YOUR SENSES/ ORGANS

You have to be aware of the senses. Your body is organically liked by external senses –

From Illness to Wellness!!!

internal organs. Your emotions will impact the external/internal organs. The expense in your externa sense such as listening, hearing beyond an upper limits will cause a distorted cell structure in external sense organ. Since, you're organically connected. Your internal organ will also be impacted.

If you practice awareness in simple things and change your ways of living..it becomes your intrinsic Nature. You've to practice as you've forgotten the language of the heart, simple alert systems. You were doing that when you were a child, and slowly you've forotton the language of the heart.

Electricy Power Station (Turbo Generator)
Well. What is the relation between the Power station your BODY? There is a correlation...

Let us say a simple example of excessive eating. We saw the process of eating, if it exceeds a specific upper limits, then it will extend its structure to adapt itself by the law of nature. Let us say a small electrical plant is capable of supplying 10MWunits of MW energy. Now, the no. of houses have increated in the locale, thus demaning more the specified upper limit of 9MW units ...you are running dangerously low. If you exceed the capacity, say it increases to 11 MWunits, then your electrical unit will run with full capacity and sometimes to the

From Illness to Wellness!!!

higher capacity to supply -2MW. In order to supply an additional capacity that was not anticipated, the accelarators producing electricity will have to extract more energy to compensate the deficit. This machine is not designed for anything beyond 10MW Production capacity. But, you've forced it to increase the supply, because the supply is more. Eventually the production unit will mal-function as you've consistently exceeded the limits. At some point, you'll need to shut-down the production unit altogether due to all mal – functioning instruments.

Now, read through the above analogy, contemplate on it by assuming the production unit as your 'sexual vital fluid' producing countless nos of prana shakthi or the life-force particles. And the instruments in the production facility are the organs internal to your body. The external senses are the consumption units such as houses with electrical gadgets using electricity. If the external conversion is higher, your external sense organs, and internal organs will start malfunction.

We have observed various healing methods of Nature. Indeed. At every step, Nature alerts you through the alert mechanism. In the above analogy of the production unit, assume an alert system. This alert system will ring every time the production capacity is increases. Then the alert system with electronic capability will do some load balancing to share the load without overloading the production unit. In similar terms, your body has alert systems in TASTE BUDS demanding a specific TASTE when the

From Illness to Wellness!!!

system is critically LOW. Or perhaps the alert symptoms of HEAD ACHE,

I request each of you to pay attention to the NATURE's alert system and heal yourself.
Guru 'Here is the souvenir' as he passes on the beautiful golden palette with the Seven Golden Rules of Wellness embossed on it.
You've mastered the Illness to Wellness program:

From Illness to Wellness;

1. Know your Anatomy;
2. Principles of Vedic Healing;
3. Transitional Therapy to Uproot your diseases ;
4. Awareness about the diseases;
5. Follow simple ways of living;
6. Healing Methods &
7. Prevention is better than cure;

Healing Meditation

I'll teach you a simple healing meditation. Aware of your breathing. Breathe in & out deeply. There is no need to hold it (2mins). Just be aware of the breathing for first couple of minutes. Then focus your attention between the eye bros on pituitary gland for couple of minutes. Visualize your body made up as millions of cells (2 mins). From there, focus your attention on the body...relax your entire body. Then, feel the Organs & say FIVE ELEMENTS are streamlined. Call out each of it "BODY-BONES (LAND), HEAT (FIRE),

From Illness to Wellness!!!

AIR, MAGNETIC ENERGY FLOW (AKASHyou're you are organically united by FIVE ELEMENTS OF NAUTRE. Every Organ is linked to the FIVE ELEMENTS. Then , visual every Organs; KIDNEY-SEX ORGAN-HEART-LUNGS-LIVER-LUNGS & external sense Organs such as EYES, EARS, NOSE & TASTE buds.

Then visualize your Organic unity with the LIFE-FORCE. There are countless no. of PRANA or LIFE FORCE in you. (energy particles). This is your ASTRAL BODY. Then, visualize your CASUAL BODY organically linked to the Cosmic consciousness. Feel blessed and bless all organisms in the WORLD. You're Organically connected.
Slowly. Descend down to the SHAKTHI KALA (starts and planets) which is the dynamic state of eternal consciousness feeling your LIFE-FORCE. Then, slowly come back to the SUN-FEEL your body, and feel your Organs. And Finally, thank them call before you conclude the meditation. You should visualize every Organ and thank them. Feel relaxed. Spend atleast 1 minute in every Organ.

Feel happy for your life & blessed.

Mr. Guru 'This is very significant and I've handed over the golden palette which will help the younger generation and many more generations to come. Go to the World and teach them about the "7 Golden Rules of Wellness". It took me more than couple of decades to master it based on my research in Eastern methods of mytics.

From Illness to Wellness!!!

I am sure this reseach will help the younger genrations to comtemplate and succeed in their endeavor. Go teach them all to transced illness and help them transfer it to wellness to lead a happy & proposerous life ahead. Dr.Ric awards him a sourvenir, a beautiful 'From Illness to Wellness' Golden palette along, with a handwritten letter.

End of Session # 14.

2025 – "WHO" Award ...
Guru's memory flashes back to the presence with the flashing cameras on stage....

Guru continues...
"Today, I am here because of this gentlemen named Dr.Raj, who is not here today to see me succeed in my endeavor. The man who showed me virtues in life by teaching the subtle techniques of 'Seven Golden Rules of Wellness'"

He shows the Golden palette to everyone in the crowd..."**From Illness to Wellness.** Today, I am standing in front of you all with confidence after achieving success in my life.

From Illness to Wellness!!!

I am honoured to indicate that I was one among the student of Maharishi, who has helped me in realizing the holistic healting methods. From that day, I had transformed from the mundane plane of life to the state of awareness. Today. It's his philosophy which is healing millions of students, and adults those who are brave enough to venture into the inner frontiers of mind.

Today, I am deeply sadened to miss my teacher, my friend, philosopher and a guide who has helped me reach here to this stage." And he paused for a while….May the soul rest in peace.

I couldn't have even moved an inch in my life without his guidance, transforming my drunken life to the Divine life of wisdom. Indeed, I am blessed to have a teacher like Dr.Raj…I salute his services to the World. The last letter from Dr. indicated these words that I cannot forget in my life time: He showcases the letter to the audience, a handwritten letter from Dr.Raj…

2005 – South Chennai.
Dear Guru,
Remember this. It's important to teach the World about the vedic healing methods which are very profound. The problem is not diseases, it's human greed and desire to commoditize diseases in the name of healthcare. You've to teach them techniques to allow Nature to heal them. There is no better Doctor than Nature. "FOOD taken in moderation is a MEDICINE" and you've to allow FIVE elements to heal you; e World on

From Illness to Wellness!!!

I felt responsible since then. My intuition based on the healing tree and Dr. Raj's support has helped me formulate these profound techniques. My goal is to teach every individual in the World to lead a healthy life. I thank you each of you for the honor. I'll not stop teaching the "Illness to Wellness" until my last breadth to heal thy World!!!

Thank you Ladies & Gentlemen!!!

From Illness to Wellness!!!

EPILOGUE

Your wellness should be the first priority. Everything else comes next. The increasing number of wellness clinics around the World has commoditized diseases. Every year the allopathic medications are released to add to your daily life. If it continues, next species that will become extinct will be the homosapiens.

You have to believe your inner self and the consciousness that is controlling as the autonomous system. Indeed, the reality is every individual is endowed with the capacity to heal thy self and there is no need for any external medications. It is your center that will guide in healing your self. Often, diseases are manifestations of your conditioned mind.

If you believe and lead a simple and profound life, Nature will heal you from within. There is no need for any external medications unless there is an absolute need depending on the situation. You're a micro-cosmic consciousness. It's your wrong behavior resulted in the diseases. The medical World is terming each of you as patients with hundreds every year. Indeed, they are like parasites sucking your blood for their survival.

The intrinsic values of your inner self and the intelligence that is taking care of you every second,

From Illness to Wellness!!!

like a mother. Do not mess up with these organs. Further, you agravate the situation by taking immediate medications. STOP DOING THAT RIGHT NOW.

You'll need to love yourself and Nature. Find ways to identify your lineage beyond the body, as you are organically connected with the whole. There is no need to be antagonistic with little symptoms of FEVER, SINUS, COUGH..which you can await for Nature to support you in the healing process. There is no need to hurry up while eating, there is a minimal process to be followed. If you do then half of these diseases will be uprooted. Then, mind should be focused towards creativity through meditative practices that will heal the connection and help you stay connected with the mother.

I request each of you contemplate on the topics, take necessary precautions to STOP unncesary medications. You must take necessary steps ahead to councel with the 'Vedic Healing' to heal yourself as discussed. This is just a beginning and a paradigm shift from the illness to the wellness.

***

From Illness to Wellness!!!

Acknowledgements

I would like to thank my family, classmates, spiritual companion and my friends, and leaders those who've inspired me without whose help this book would never have been completed.

I'd like to thank Dr. Madhavan (CEO, BIST), Sukumar Subramanian (CEO, VMG Entertainment, India), Chandrasekar Papudesu, MIT, US (Director, IBM US) & Louis Victor Jayaraj (Sr.Director, Huawei India Technologies Ltd) for their valuable feedback and suggestions to improve the manuscript.

Thank you for your patience and guidance… *The references to the healing techniques are taught in "Anatomy Therapy" sessions conductd by Healer. Bhaskar. Thank you sir!*

www.ingramcontent.com/pod-product-compliance
Lightning Source LLC
Chambersburg PA
CBHW051704170526
45167CB00002B/531